CNA
SIMPLIFIED
QUESTIONS & ANSWERS

EDGAR G. KARLSSON

Copyright © 2024 by EDGAR G. KARLSSON

All rights reserved.

DISCLAIMER

The information contained in this book is intended solely for educational and informational purposes to assist individuals in preparing for the Certified Nursing Assistant (CNA) examination. While every effort has been made to ensure the accuracy and completeness of the material presented, this book is not intended to serve as a substitute for professional medical advice, diagnosis, or treatment.

TABLE OF CONTENTS

INTRODUCTION .... Error! Bookmark not defined.

Disclaimer 3

INTRODUCTION 5

Purpose of the Guide 5

What is a Certified Nursing Assistant? 5

Overview of the CNA Exam 6

CHPTHER ONE 7

CHAPTER TWO 37

CHAPTER THREE 64

CHAPTER FOUR 96

CHAPTER FIVE 120

CHAPTHER SIX..Error! Bookmark not defined.

INTRODUCTION

Welcome to the Certified Nursing Assistant (CNA) Exam Preparation Guide. This book is designed to support you on your journey to becoming a Certified Nursing Assistant, offering you the knowledge, skills, and confidence needed to excel in both the CNA exam and your future career.

Purpose of the Guide

The primary purpose of this guide is to provide a comprehensive resource for individuals preparing to take the CNA certification exam. The CNA exam is a crucial step in your career as it validates your ability to provide quality care to patients in various healthcare settings. This guide aims to:

- **Enhance Your Knowledge**: Cover essential concepts in patient care, clinical skills, and healthcare regulations.
- **Improve Your Skills**: Offer practical tips and techniques for performing key clinical tasks and procedures.
- **Boost Your Confidence**: Prepare you for both the written and skills components of the CNA exam with practice questions, sample tests, and test-taking strategies.

What is a Certified Nursing Assistant?

A Certified Nursing Assistant (CNA) plays a vital role in the healthcare system, offering direct care and support to patients under the supervision of registered nurses (RNs) and licensed practical nurses (LPNs). CNAs work in various settings, including hospitals, nursing homes, assisted living facilities, and home care environments. Their responsibilities include:

- **Personal Care**: Assisting patients with activities of daily living such as bathing, dressing, and grooming.
- **Vital Signs Monitoring**: Measuring and recording vital signs like blood pressure, pulse, respiration, and temperature.
- **Mobility Assistance**: Helping patients with mobility, including transferring from bed to chair and walking.
- **Communication**: Providing emotional support and effective communication with patients and their families.

Overview of the CNA Exam

The CNA exam is designed to evaluate your knowledge and practical skills necessary for effective patient care. The exam typically consists of two main components:

- **Written Test**: This part of the exam assesses your understanding of nursing concepts, patient care procedures, and healthcare regulations through multiple-choice questions. It covers topics such as infection control, patient rights, and emergency procedures.
- **Skills Test**: The skills test evaluates your ability to perform specific clinical tasks. You will be required to demonstrate competency in skills such as taking vital signs, assisting with personal care, and implementing safety measures. This part of the exam is conducted in a hands-on, practical setting.

CHPTHER ONE

QUESTION AND ANSWERS

1. What is the normal range for an adult's body temperature in Fahrenheit?

A) 96.8 - 98.6

B) 97.8 - 99.0

C) 98.6 - 100.4

D) 99.0 - 100.8

2. Which of the following is a sign of infection?

A) Decreased appetite

B) Decreased urination

C) Elevated temperature

D) Normal blood pressure

3. What is the primary purpose of hand hygiene in healthcare?

A) To prevent the spread of germs and infections

B) To keep hands soft and moisturized

C) To remove visible dirt and grime

D) To improve patient comfort

4. When assisting a patient with mobility, which of the following should be prioritized?

A) The patient's comfort

B) The patient's safety

C) The speed of the transfer

D) The convenience for the healthcare worker

5. What does the acronym "RACE" stand for in fire safety protocols?

A) Rescue, Alarm, Contain, Extinguish

B) Rescue, Alarm, Clear, Evacuate

C) Rescue, Assess, Contain, Exit

D) Respond, Alarm, Contain, Evacuate

6. What is the normal range for an adult's resting pulse rate?

A) 40 - 60 beats per minute

B) 60 - 100 beats per minute

C) 100 - 120 beats per minute

D) 120 - 140 beats per minute

7. Which position is best for a patient experiencing difficulty breathing?

A) Supine

B) Prone

C) Fowler's

D) Trendelenburg

8. What is the correct method for measuring blood pressure?

A) Use a sphygmomanometer and stethoscope on the wrist

B) Use a digital monitor on the upper arm

C) Use a sphygmomanometer and stethoscope on the upper arm

D) Use a digital monitor on the lower leg

9. Which of the following should be done first when a patient falls?

A) Move the patient to a safe location

B) Check the patient's vital signs

C) Call for help

D) Document the incident

10. What is the primary purpose of using personal protective equipment (PPE)?

A) To protect the healthcare worker from physical injury

B) To protect the patient from infection

C) To ensure compliance with healthcare regulations

D) To maintain a clean working environment

11. How often should a patient's vital signs be checked in a stable condition?

A) Every 15 minutes

B) Every 30 minutes

C) Every hour

D) Every 4 to 8 hours

12. What is the best way to prevent the spread of respiratory infections?

A) Regular hand washing

B) Wearing gloves

C) Using hand sanitizer

D) Wearing masks only

13. What is the purpose of a bed rail?

A) To keep the bed clean

B) To assist the patient in getting up

C) To prevent the patient from falling out of bed

D) To enhance the aesthetic of the room

14. What should a CNA do if a patient complains of chest pain?

A) Administer medication as needed

B) Perform a thorough physical examination

C) Inform the nurse or physician immediately

D) Reassure the patient and monitor

15. Which of the following is a key component of patient privacy?

A) Discussing patient information only with authorized personnel

B) Sharing patient information with family members

C) Posting patient information on the bulletin board

D) Using social media to discuss patient care

16. When assisting a patient with feeding, what is the best practice?

A) Provide food and drink in large portions

B) Allow the patient to eat at their own pace and preferences

C) Feed the patient quickly to save time

D) Encourage the patient to eat a specific amount

17. What is the normal range for an adult's respiratory rate?

A) 10 - 20 breaths per minute

B) 20 - 30 breaths per minute

C) 30 - 40 breaths per minute

D) 40 - 50 breaths per minute

18. What should a CNA do if they notice a change in a patient's mental status?

    A) Document the change and continue monitoring

    B) Ignore the change if the patient is stable

    C) Report the change to the nurse or physician immediately

E) Ask the patient if they feel different

19. Which of the following is a proper method for taking a patient's oral temperature?

    A) Place the thermometer under the armpit

    B) Place the thermometer in the rectum

    C) Place the thermometer in the mouth, under the tongue

    D) Place the thermometer in the ear canal

20. What is the primary goal of patient positioning?

    A) To enhance patient comfort and satisfaction

    B) To facilitate patient mobility and ease of access for healthcare providers

    C) To prevent complications such as pressure ulcers and improve circulation

    D) To meet healthcare facility standards

21. What is the correct technique for performing hand hygiene?

    A) Use soap and water, rubbing hands for at least 20 seconds

    B) Use hand sanitizer for 10 seconds

    C) Wash hands under running water for 10 seconds

D) Use alcohol wipes for 30 seconds

22. When should a CNA use gloves?

A) Only when performing invasive procedures

B) Only when handling food

C) When coming into contact with blood or body fluids

D) Only when cleaning the patient's room

23. How should a CNA handle a patient with a known allergy to latex?

A) Use latex gloves for all procedures

B) Avoid using latex products and use alternative materials

C) Ask the patient to wear a latex allergy bracelet

D) Inform the patient they need to manage their allergy themselves

24. What should a CNA do if they notice a patient's wound is bleeding profusely?

A) Apply pressure to the wound and call for help

B) Clean the wound and apply a bandage

C) Ignore the bleeding and monitor the patient

D) Change the wound dressing

25. How should a CNA address a patient's request for assistance with personal hygiene?

A) Provide the assistance as quickly as possible to avoid delays

B) Ask the patient to wait until it is convenient for you

C) Explain the procedure and provide assistance promptly

D) Direct the patient to perform personal hygiene independently

26. Which of the following is an important aspect of patient documentation?

   A) Include personal opinions about the patient's behavior

   B) Use clear, concise, and objective language

   C) Document only significant changes in the patient's condition

   D) Write in a subjective manner to provide detailed descriptions

27. What is the proper technique for transferring a patient from a bed to a wheelchair?

   A) Lift the patient directly without assistance

   B) Use a transfer belt and maintain proper body mechanics

   C) Drag the patient across the bed

   D) Use a mechanical lift without assistance

28. What should a CNA do if a patient is having a seizure?

   A) Restrain the patient to prevent injury

   B) Place a pillow under the patient's head and keep them safe

   C) Leave the patient alone to recover

   D) Administer medication immediately

29. What is the main purpose of the Fowler's position?

   A) To promote comfort and aid in digestion

   B) To assist in breathing and improve circulation

   C) To help with gastrointestinal issues

   D) To prevent pressure ulcers

30. How should a CNA respond to a patient who is anxious about an upcoming procedure?

A) Ignore their concerns and proceed with the procedure

B) Provide reassurance and explain the procedure clearly

C) Tell the patient to be calm and not worry

D) Rush through the procedure to minimize their anxiety

31. What is the normal range for an adult's blood pressure?

A) 90/60 mmHg - 120/80 mmHg

B) 100/70 mmHg - 130/90 mmHg

C) 110/80 mmHg - 140/100 mmHg

D) 120/80 mmHg - 150/100 mmHg

32. What is the correct way to measure a patient's weight?

A) Ask the patient to step on the scale without shoes

B) Measure the patient's weight while they are seated

C) Use a tape measure to estimate weight

D) Measure the patient's weight at the same time each day

33. How should a CNA handle a patient who refuses to take medication?

A) Force the medication into the patient's mouth

B) Respect the patient's decision and inform the nurse

C) Ignore the refusal and document the medication administration

E) Ask the patient to reconsider and provide additional information

34. What is an important consideration when providing catheter care?

A) Clean the catheter with soap and water only

B) Keep the catheter tubing above the level of the bladder

C) Change the catheter daily

D) Remove the catheter if it becomes uncomfortable

35. What does the term "standard precautions" refer to in healthcare settings?

A) Measures to prevent the spread of infections through blood and body fluids

B) Guidelines for the use of personal protective equipment only

C) Procedures for handling medical waste and sharps

D) Practices for ensuring patient comfort and satisfaction

36. When should a CNA report a change in a patient's condition to a nurse?

A) Only if the change is severe or life-threatening

B) Whenever there is a noticeable change, regardless of severity

C) After documenting the change in the patient's chart

D) At the end of the shift during handover

37. What is the purpose of using assistive devices such as walkers and canes?

A) To enhance patient mobility and provide support

B) To replace the need for physical therapy

C) To prevent patient falls by restricting movement

D) To assist healthcare workers in moving patients

38. What should be done if a CNA accidentally spills a hazardous substance?

A) Clean up the spill immediately with available supplies

B) Inform the nurse and follow the facility's protocol for spill management

C) Ignore the spill if it is minor

E) Ask the patient to clean up the spill

39. What is the best practice for maintaining patient privacy during care?

A) Use privacy curtains and ensure doors are closed

B) Discuss patient information openly with colleagues

C) Leave the patient's information visible on the desk

D) Post patient details on the notice board for staff to see

40. How should a CNA assist a patient with a mobility impairment when using the toilet?

A) Assist the patient without providing privacy

B) Provide assistance and ensure the patient's dignity and privacy

C) Leave the patient alone and monitor from outside the bathroom

D) Use a bedpan or commode without explanation

41. What is the purpose of using a transfer belt?

A) To provide a secure way to lift and move patients

B) To prevent patients from falling out of bed

C) To assist with daily hygiene routines

D) To secure patients during medical procedure

42. Which of the following is a common symptom of dehydration?

A) Weight gain

B) Moist skin

C) Dry mouth and skin

D) Increased urination

43. What is the best practice for providing post-operative care?

A) Monitor the patient for complications and provide comfort measures

B) Allow the patient to rest without monitoring

C) Provide extensive explanations about the surgery

D) Ignore any signs of discomfort unless specifically mentioned by the patient

44. How should a CNA approach a patient with a known cognitive impairment?

A) Use clear, simple instructions and be patient

B) Speak quickly and use complex language

C) Avoid interaction and focus on other tasks

D) Use a stern tone to encourage compliance

45. What is the correct procedure for disposing of sharps?

A) Place them in a regular trash can

B) Dispose of them in a designated sharps container

C) Flush them down the toilet

D) Recycle them with other medical waste

46. What should a CNA do if a patient experiences sudden shortness of breath?

A) Reassure the patient and continue monitoring

B) Assist the patient into a comfortable position and call for medical help

C) Administer medication as per the patient's previous orders

D) Ignore the symptoms and document the event

47. What is the primary reason for performing regular repositioning of bedridden patients?

A) To prevent pressure ulcers and improve circulation

B) To enhance patient comfort and avoid boredom

C) To facilitate easier patient access for healthcare workers

D) To promote patient participation in care

48. How should a CNA handle a patient who is verbally aggressive?

A) Respond aggressively to maintain authority

B) Remain calm and try to de-escalate the situation

C) Ignore the aggression and continue with care

D) Report the aggression to family members immediately

49. What is the purpose of using a bedpan?

A) To provide a comfortable place for patients to rest

B) To assist patients with urinary and bowel elimination

C) To prevent patients from using the bathroom

D) To facilitate personal hygiene

50. What should a CNA do if they notice a patient's blood pressure is elevated?

A) Take the blood pressure again and report the findings to the nurse

B) Document the elevated blood pressure and continue monitoring

C) Reassure the patient without taking further action

D) Administer blood pressure medication as needed

51. Which position is used to enhance comfort for a patient with abdominal pain?

   A) Supine

   B) Prone

   C) Fowler's

   D) Side-lying

52. What is the best way to prevent the spread of gastrointestinal infections?

   A) Using proper hand hygiene and sanitizing surfaces

   B) Wearing personal protective equipment only

   C) Avoiding patient contact altogether

   D) Using disposable utensils for all patients

53. What is the appropriate action if a CNA suspects a patient is being abused?

   A) Document the suspicions and report to the nurse or appropriate authority

   B) Confront the suspected abuser directly

   C) Ignore the suspicions unless evidence is clear

   D) Discuss the situation with other staff members

54. How should a CNA manage a patient with an indwelling catheter?

A) Ensure the catheter is secured and the drainage bag is below the level of the bladder

B) Remove and clean the catheter daily

C) Replace the catheter if there is any discomfort

D) Allow the patient to manage the catheter themselves

55. What is the purpose of providing emotional support to patients?

A) To enhance patient satisfaction and comfort

B) To encourage patients to follow treatment plans

C) To build rapport and improve communication

D) To distract patients from their physical symptoms

56. What is the correct technique for measuring a patient's height?

A) Measure while the patient is lying down

B) Measure while the patient is seated

C) Measure while the patient is standing with heels together

D) Measure while the patient is in a wheelchair

57. What is the purpose of a medical alert bracelet?

A) To provide emergency contact information

B) To inform healthcare providers of specific medical conditions or allergies

C) To enhance the patient's overall appearance

D) To indicate the patient's insurance provider

58. When should a CNA perform patient care tasks?

A) Only during scheduled care times

B) Based on the patient's needs and care plan

C) At the convenience of the CNA

D) After completing all other tasks for the day

59. How should a CNA handle a situation where a patient is incontinent?

A) Assist the patient with changing and ensure they are comfortable and clean

B) Ask the patient to manage their incontinence independently

C) Ignore the situation if the patient is not complaining

D) Document the incident and proceed with other tasks

60. What is the most important consideration when providing care to a patient with diabetes?

A) Monitoring blood glucose levels and providing appropriate care

B) Limiting the patient's food intake to avoid complications

C) Ensuring the patient follows a strict diet without deviation

D) Avoiding all physical activity to prevent blood sugar spikes

61. What is a key component of effective patient communication?

A) Using medical jargon to ensure accuracy

B) Speaking clearly and listening actively

C) Asking closed-ended questions for quick responses

D) Providing minimal information to save time

62. How should a CNA address a patient who is experiencing nausea?

A) Offer the patient a drink of water and wait for symptoms to pass

B) Inform the nurse and provide comfort measures as appropriate

C) Administer anti-nausea medication without notifying the nurse

D) Encourage the patient to eat small meals frequently

63. What should a CNA do if they notice a patient is showing signs of severe dehydration?

A) Provide fluids and monitor the patient closely

B) Administer intravenous fluids as needed

C) Notify the nurse or physician immediately

D) Allow the patient to drink fluids at their own pace

64. What is the best practice for using a gait belt?

A) Secure the belt around the patient's waist and provide support during ambulation

B) Use the gait belt only for lifting patients

C) Place the gait belt loosely around the patient's hips

D) Remove the gait belt once the patient is standing

65. How should a CNA handle a patient's request for privacy?

A) Close curtains and doors as needed to respect the patient's privacy

B) Tell the patient to wait until the end of your shift for privacy

C) Discuss the patient's needs with other staff members openly

D) Ignore the request if it is not feasible at the moment

66. What is the primary goal of patient care planning?

A) To outline specific interventions and goals for the patient's care

B) To provide a schedule for healthcare providers

C) To document patient progress for legal purposes

D) To establish a routine for the CNA's daily tasks

67. What is the proper procedure for applying a new bandage to a wound?

A) Clean the wound, apply a sterile bandage, and secure it in place

B) Apply ointment to the wound before placing the bandage

C) Use non-sterile materials and cover the wound loosely

D) Apply a bandage without cleaning the wound first

68. How should a CNA handle a patient who is experiencing severe pain?

A) Provide comfort measures and notify the nurse or physician immediately

B) Ignore the pain if it seems manageable

C) Administer pain medication as per the patient's request

D) Tell the patient to rest and avoid discussing the pain

69. What is the correct technique for using a thermometer to measure an axillary temperature?

A) Place the thermometer under the patient's arm and hold it in place for the recommended time

B) Insert the thermometer into the patient's mouth and close the lips around it

C) Place the thermometer in the patient's rectum for a more accurate reading

D) Place the thermometer in the patient's ear canal

70. What is an important consideration when assisting a patient with feeding?

A) Ensuring the patient is in an upright position and offering small, manageable portions

B) Encouraging the patient to eat quickly to complete the meal

C) Providing large portions to ensure adequate nutrition

D) Feeding the patient without checking for any food allergies

71. What is the appropriate action when a patient expresses fear or anxiety about a procedure?

A) Address their concerns, provide reassurance, and explain the procedure clearly

B) Ignore their concerns and proceed with the procedure

C) Tell them to be calm and avoid discussing their fears

D) Rush through the procedure to minimize their anxiety

72. What is the main purpose of using a pressure-relief device for a bedridden patient?

A) To prevent the development of pressure ulcers and promote skin health

B) To enhance the patient's comfort and provide additional cushioning

C) To facilitate easier patient repositioning and mobility

D) To provide a more aesthetically pleasing bed setup

73. What should a CNA do if a patient exhibits signs of a stroke?

A) Perform a quick assessment and notify emergency medical services immediately

B) Provide the patient with water and wait for symptoms to improve

C) Document the symptoms and continue monitoring the patient

D) Administer medication if the patient has a prescription

74. What is the correct technique for performing a wound dressing change?

A) Use sterile gloves and clean the wound with an appropriate solution before applying a new dressing

B) Change the dressing without cleaning the wound

C) Use non-sterile gloves and apply a new dressing

D) Clean the wound and apply a dressing without gloves

75. How should a CNA respond to a patient who is confused and disoriented?

A) Speak clearly and calmly, and provide reassurance

B) Ignore the confusion and continue with routine tasks

C) Raise your voice to get the patient's attention

D) Provide complex explanations to clarify the situation

76. What is the proper method for documenting patient care?

A) Use objective, clear, and concise language

B) Include personal opinions and subjective statements

C) Document only the major events and changes

D) Avoid writing details about routine care

77. What should a CNA do if they notice a patient has difficulty breathing?

A) Assist the patient into a comfortable position and call for help

B) Provide the patient with a warm blanket and wait

C) Administer oxygen if available and appropriate

D) Ignore the difficulty and monitor the patient

78. How should a CNA handle a situation where a patient's family member is being disruptive?

A) Address the family member calmly and involve them in the care process

B) Ignore the disruption and continue with patient care

C) Ask the family member to leave the facility immediately

D) Report the disruption to the nursing supervisor

79. What is the purpose of using a surgical mask in healthcare settings?

A) To protect the patient from respiratory droplets

B) To maintain personal hygiene

C) To ensure compliance with dress code regulations

D) To enhance communication with the patient

80. How should a CNA approach a patient with limited English proficiency?

A) Use simple language and gestures, and consider using an interpreter if available

B) Speak quickly and use medical terminology

C) Ignore the language barrier and continue with care

D) Provide written instructions only

81. What is the correct action if a patient's blood glucose level is too high?

A) Notify the nurse or physician and follow their instructions

B) Provide the patient with additional insulin immediately

C) Ignore the reading if the patient feels fine

D) Recheck the blood glucose level and document the results

82. How should a CNA handle a patient who is exhibiting signs of an allergic reaction?

A) Monitor the patient's symptoms and notify the nurse or physician immediately

B) Ignore the symptoms and provide comfort measures

C) Administer allergy medication as per the patient's request

D) Ask the patient to manage the reaction themselves

83. What is the best practice for ensuring patient safety during a bath or shower?

A) Provide non-slip mats and assist the patient as needed

B) Allow the patient to bathe independently without supervision

C) Use hot water to ensure the patient is comfortable

D) Rush the bathing process to save time

84. What is the main purpose of patient education?

A) To empower patients to manage their own health and care

B) To complete required paperwork and documentation

C) To provide entertainment and distraction for patients

D) To ensure patients follow strict healthcare protocols

85. How should a CNA respond to a patient with a pressure ulcer?

A) Provide appropriate wound care and notify the nurse

B) Ignore the ulcer and document the occurrence

C) Apply over-the-counter ointments without consulting the nurse

D) Avoid discussing the ulcer with the patient

86. What is the correct procedure for handling soiled linens?

A) Place them in a designated linen hamper or bag immediately

B) Leave them on the floor until the end of the shift

C) Wash them in the patient's room

D) Reuse them after shaking them out

87. How should a CNA assist a patient who is experiencing a urinary tract infection?

    A) Encourage fluid intake and monitor symptoms

    B) Administer antibiotics without medical orders

    C) Provide a catheter for continuous drainage

    D) Ignore the symptoms and document the infection

88. What is an important aspect of caring for a patient with a wound drain?

    A) Monitor the drain for proper function and report any issues

    B) Remove the drain if it becomes uncomfortable for the patient

    C) Clean the drain with non-sterile solutions

    D) Avoid touching the drain to prevent contamination

89. What should a CNA do if a patient reports feeling faint or dizzy?

    A) Assist the patient to a safe position and monitor closely

    B) Provide the patient with food and drink immediately

    C) Ignore the symptoms and continue with care

D) Document the symptoms and inform the family

90. How should a CNA handle a situation where a patient's family member requests confidential information?

A) Explain that you cannot provide information without patient consent

B) Share the information if you believe it is in the patient's best interest

C) Provide the information to maintain family trust

D) Refer the family member to the healthcare provider

91. What is the purpose of providing range-of-motion exercises?

A) To maintain joint flexibility and prevent contractures

B) To enhance muscle strength and endurance

C) To reduce the need for physical therapy

D) To improve the patient's overall comfort

92. How should a CNA manage a patient who is at risk for falls?

A) Ensure the environment is free of hazards and use assistive devices as needed

B) Restrict the patient's mobility to prevent falls

C) Provide the patient with a fall alert bracelet only

D) Ignore the risk and monitor the patient

93. What is the correct way to measure a patient's fluid intake?

A) Record all fluids consumed, including water, juices, and soups

B) Only record fluids provided by healthcare staff

C) Estimate fluid intake based on visual observation

D) Measure only fluids consumed during meal times

94. How should a CNA assist a patient who is bedridden and experiencing constipation?

A) Provide a high-fiber diet, encourage fluids, and assist with bowel routines

B) Administer laxatives without consulting the nurse

C) Avoid discussing bowel habits with the patient

D) Encourage the patient to rest and avoid dietary changes

95. What is the purpose of using anti-embolic stockings?

A) To prevent blood clots and promote circulation in the legs

B) To provide additional comfort and warmth to the legs

C) To restrict movement and prevent falls

D) To enhance the appearance of the patient's legs

96. How should a CNA respond if a patient expresses concerns about their treatment plan?

A) Listen to their concerns and discuss them with the healthcare team

B) Dismiss their concerns and proceed with the current plan

C) Reassure them without making any changes to the treatment plan

D) Change the treatment plan based on the patient's request

97. What is an important consideration when providing care to a patient with a mental health condition?

A) Approach the patient with empathy and understanding, and respect their individuality

B) Avoid discussing their condition to prevent worsening symptoms

C) Use authoritative language to ensure compliance with treatment

D) Focus solely on physical care and ignore mental health needs

98. How should a CNA address a patient's concerns about their medication?

A) Notify the nurse or pharmacist to address the concerns

B) Change the medication based on the patient's request

C) Ignore the concerns if they seem minor

D) Provide the medication without discussing it with the patient

99. What is the correct way to measure a patient's weight?

A) Use a calibrated scale and ensure the patient is in a consistent state (e.g., minimal clothing, no shoes)

B) Estimate weight based on previous records and visual assessment

C) Measure weight at irregular intervals throughout the day

D) Use a bed scale without accounting for the patient's position

100. How should a CNA assist a patient with mobility challenges in transferring from bed to wheelchair?

A) Use proper body mechanics and assistive devices, and ensure patient safety during the transfer

B) Lift the patient manually to avoid using assistive devices

C) Allow the patient to transfer independently to encourage self-reliance

D) Skip the transfer if the patient seems uncomfortable

ANSWERS

1. A)	26. A)	51. D)	76. A)
2. B)	27. A)	52. A)	77. A)
3. A)	28. A)	53. A)	78. A)
4. A)	29. B)	54. A)	79. A)
5. A)	30. A)	55. A)	80. A)
6. B)	31. B)	56. C)	81. A)
7. A)	32. B)	57. B)	82. A)
8. A)	33. D)	58. B)	83. A)
9. A)	34. B)	59. A)	84. A)
10. A)	35. A)	60. A)	85. A)
11. B)	36. B)	61. B)	86. A)
12. A)	37. A)	62. B)	87. A)
13. A)	38. B)	63. C)	88. A)
14. A)	39. A)	64. A)	89. A)
15. A)	40. B)	65. A)	90. A)
16. A)	41. A)	66. A)	91. A)
17. A)	42. C)	67. A)	92. A)
18. B)	43. A)	68. A)	93. A)
19. A)	44. A)	69. A)	94. A)
20. A)	45. B)	70. A)	95. A)
21. A)	46. B)	71. A)	96. A)
22. A)	47. A)	72. A)	97. A)
23. B)	48. B)	73. A)	98. A)
24. A)	49. B)	74. A)	99. A)
25. A)	50. A)	75. A)	100. A)

CHAPTER TWO

QUESTION AND ANSWER

1. What is the first step in handwashing according to standard procedures?

   A) Apply soap to dry hands

   B) Wet hands with warm water

   C) Dry hands with a clean towel

   D) Rub hands together with soap

2. When performing a blood pressure measurement, which artery should the cuff be placed over?

   A) Femoral artery

   B) Brachial artery

   C) Radial artery

   D) Carotid artery

3. How often should vital signs be checked for a stable patient in a routine hospital setting?

   A) Every 15 minutes

   B) Every 30 minutes

C) Every 1-2 hours

D) Every 4-8 hours

4. What position is typically used for abdominal examinations?

    A) Supine

    B) Prone

    C) Lateral

    D) Fowler's

5. What is the purpose of using a transfer belt during patient transfers?

    A) To enhance patient comfort

    B) To prevent falls and ensure safety

    C) To restrict patient movement

    D) To provide a secure way to lift patients

6. When administering oral medications, which of the following is a key safety step?

    A) Ensure the patient is sitting upright

    B) Crush all medications to facilitate swallowing

    C) Administer medications without checking the patient's identity

D) Use a medication cup for all types of medications

7. How should a CNA correctly measure a patient's temperature using a digital thermometer?

A) Place the thermometer under the patient's tongue for oral temperature

B) Insert the thermometer into the patient's rectum for rectal temperature

C) Place the thermometer under the patient's armpit for axillary temperature

D) Insert the thermometer into the patient's ear for tympanic temperature

8. What is the proper technique for making an occupied bed?

A) Remove all linens at once and then replace with new linens

B) Change the linens while the patient is in the bed, rolling the old linens to one side

C) Remove linens and immediately place new linens without touching the patient

D) Change linens while the patient is out of the bed

9. Which position is recommended for a patient experiencing shortness of breath?

A) Supine

B) Prone

C) Fowler's

D) Trendelenburg

10. How should a CNA handle a patient who has a nasogastric (NG) tube?

A) Flush the tube with water before and after feeding

B) Avoid touching the tube to prevent contamination

C) Clamp the tube during meals to avoid leakage

D) Remove the tube if the patient complains of discomfort

11. What is the purpose of using a bedpan?

A) To assist patients with urinary and bowel elimination

B) To provide support for sitting up in bed

C) To elevate the patient's legs during rest

D) To collect specimens for laboratory analysis

12. What should a CNA do if they discover a patient has an open wound?

A) Clean the wound with soap and water and apply a sterile dressing

B) Leave the wound uncovered and report it to the nurse

C) Apply an over-the-counter ointment and bandage it

D) Cover the wound with a non-sterile cloth and report it

13. When using a gait belt, where should it be positioned on the patient?

A) Around the patient's chest

B) Across the patient's abdomen

C) Around the patient's waist

D) Under the patient's arms

14. What is the primary purpose of range-of-motion (ROM) exercises?

A) To enhance muscle strength and endurance

B) To prevent joint stiffness and maintain flexibility

C) To increase the patient's appetite

D) To improve cardiovascular health

15. How should a CNA handle soiled linens?

A) Place them in a designated linen hamper immediately

B) Fold and store them until the end of the shift

C) Dispose of them in the patient's room trash can

D) Reuse them after washing with disinfectant

16. What is the appropriate method for measuring a patient's pulse?

A) Use a sphygmomanometer to measure pulse rate

B) Palpate the pulse at the wrist or neck and count beats per minute

C) Use an electronic thermometer to measure pulse rate

D) Listen to the pulse using a stethoscope at the patient's chest

17. When performing catheter care, what should a CNA do to prevent infection?

A) Clean the catheter and surrounding area with soap and water

B) Change the catheter daily to avoid infection

C) Leave the catheter uncovered to ensure ventilation

D) Use non-sterile wipes to clean the catheter

18. How should a CNA position a patient who is unconscious and requires frequent repositioning?

A) Reposition the patient every 2 hours to prevent pressure ulcers

B) Reposition the patient only when signs of discomfort are observed

C) Reposition the patient every 4 hours to ensure comfort

D) Allow the patient to remain in one position for comfort

19. What is the correct procedure for assisting a patient with a feeding tube?

A) Ensure the patient is in an upright position and verify tube placement

B) Administer the feed while the patient is lying flat in bed

C) Flush the tube with water only after feeding is completed

D) Discontinue the feeding if the patient shows any signs of discomfort

20. How should a CNA respond if a patient refuses to take their medication?

A) Report the refusal to the nurse and document the incident

B) Administer the medication anyway to ensure compliance

C) Force the medication into the patient's mouth

D) Ignore the refusal if the medication is not critical

21. What is the most important aspect of using an oxygen mask with a patient?

A) Ensure the mask fits snugly over the patient's nose and mouth

B) Remove the mask if the patient feels uncomfortable

C) Adjust the oxygen flow based on the patient's request

D) Use the mask only during sleep

22. When taking an axillary temperature, how long should the thermometer be left in place?

A) 1-2 minutes

B) 3-4 minutes

C) 5-6 minutes

D) 7-8 minutes

23. What is the primary goal of performing hand hygiene?

A) To reduce the risk of spreading infections

B) To keep hands smelling pleasant

C) To maintain skin moisture and prevent dryness

E) To ensure hands are free from visible dirt

24. What should a CNA do if they notice that a patient has a sudden change in mental status?

A) Report the change immediately to the nurse

B) Document the change and monitor the patient closely

C) Administer medication as prescribed to address the change

D) Ignore the change if the patient is stable otherwise

25. How should a CNA properly assist a patient with a walker?

A) Ensure the walker is within reach and the patient is stable before walking

B) Push the walker for the patient to ensure proper movement

C) Allow the patient to use the walker independently without supervision

D) Remove the walker if the patient feels it is hindering their mobility

26. What is the correct technique for measuring a patient's respiration rate?

A) Count the number of breaths for 30 seconds and multiply by 2

B) Observe the chest rise and fall for 1 minute

C) Measure respiration while the patient is talking

D) Use a stethoscope to listen for breath sounds for 5 minutes

27. What should a CNA do when assisting with a bed bath?

A) Ensure the patient is comfortable and provide privacy during the bath

B) Use a single cloth for the entire bath to conserve resources

C) Perform the bath quickly to minimize patient discomfort

D) Avoid using soap to prevent skin irritation

28. How should a CNA handle a patient who is at risk of falling?

A) Ensure the environment is free of hazards and assist with mobility

B) Restrict the patient's movements to prevent falls

C) Use restraints to keep the patient safe

D) Avoid providing assistance to encourage independence

29. What is the appropriate method for taking a radial pulse?

A) Place fingers on the patient's wrist and count beats for 1 minute

B) Place fingers on the patient's neck and count beats for 30 seconds

C) Use a stethoscope on the patient's chest and count beats for 1 minute

D) Count beats for 15 seconds and multiply by 4

30. How should a CNA handle a patient with incontinence?

A) Provide regular toileting and use absorbent products as needed

B) Restrict fluid intake to reduce incontinence

C) Leave the patient in wet linens until they are dry

D) Administer medications to control incontinence

31. When performing oral care for an unconscious patient, what should a CNA do?

A) Position the patient on their side and use a sponge to clean the mouth

B) Brush the patient's teeth as you would for a conscious patient

C) Use mouthwash and avoid brushing the teeth

D) Clean the mouth with a dry cloth

32. How should a CNA assist a patient with a mechanical lift?

A) Ensure the patient is securely strapped and lift them slowly

B) Lift the patient without strapping them to avoid discomfort

C) Use the lift only if the patient requests it

D) Allow the patient to operate the lift independently

33. What is the purpose of using a TED hose?

A) To prevent blood clots and promote circulation in the legs

B) To provide warmth and comfort to the legs

C) To support the patient's knees during movement

D) To improve skin appearance and reduce swelling

34. What should a CNA do if a patient exhibits signs of an allergic reaction?

A) Report the symptoms to the nurse immediately and document them

B) Administer an antihistamine without consulting a nurse

C) Ignore the symptoms if the patient seems stable

D) Reassure the patient and wait for the reaction to subside

35. When assisting a patient with eating, what is an important consideration?

A) Ensure the patient is in an upright position and offer small, manageable portions

B) Encourage the patient to eat quickly to complete the meal

C) Feed the patient without asking for their preferences

D) Use a spoon for all types of food regardless of texture

36. How should a CNA perform an assessment of a patient's skin?

A) Observe for any changes in color, temperature, and texture

B) Only check the skin if the patient complains of discomfort

C) Inspect the skin only in areas exposed to the sun

D) Avoid touching the skin to prevent causing discomfort

37. What is the correct way to perform a manual blood glucose test?

A) Cleanse the finger with alcohol, prick with a lancet, and apply blood to the test strip

B) Use a needle to draw blood from the patient's vein

C) Apply the glucose meter to the patient's arm for a reading

D) Collect urine samples for glucose testing

38. What should a CNA do if a patient is having difficulty breathing?

A) Place the patient in an upright position and call for medical assistance

B) Administer oxygen without consulting a nurse

C) Reassure the patient and avoid checking vital signs

D) Ignore the symptoms if the patient is alert and conscious

39. When performing a dressing change, what is the most important step?

A) Wash hands thoroughly and use sterile equipment

B) Apply the dressing without cleaning the wound

C) Change the dressing quickly to minimize discomfort

D) Leave the wound uncovered to air out

40. How should a CNA assist a patient with a hip replacement?

A) Follow the healthcare provider's instructions on movement and positioning

B) Encourage the patient to bend and twist at the hip as much as possible

C) Allow the patient to walk without any assistance

D) Reposition the patient frequently to prevent stiffness

41. What is the correct procedure for measuring a patient's height?

A) Have the patient stand on a flat surface and use a measuring tape

B) Measure the patient's height while seated in a wheelchair

C) Measure the patient's height while lying in bed

D) Use a wall-mounted stadiometer and have the patient stand straight

42. What should a CNA do if a patient is experiencing nausea?

A) Offer a basin for vomiting and report the symptoms to the nurse

B) Provide the patient with solid food to settle their stomach

C) Ignore the symptoms if the patient is not in pain

D) Administer anti-nausea medication without a prescription

43. How should a CNA perform a urinary catheter insertion?

A) Follow sterile technique and ensure proper placement

B) Insert the catheter using clean gloves and a non-sterile technique

C) Insert the catheter without any lubrication to avoid discomfort

D) Use a pre-filled catheter and avoid using any sterile supplies

44. What is the proper method for measuring an infant's weight?

A) Use an infant scale and ensure the infant is undressed for accuracy

B) Weigh the infant while holding them and subtract your weight

C) Use a standard scale and estimate the infant's weight

D) Weigh the infant while they are in their crib

45. When assisting with a tracheostomy, what is an essential step?

A) Ensure the tracheostomy tube is clear and the area around it is clean

B) Remove the tracheostomy tube if the patient is having difficulty breathing

C) Use non-sterile equipment to clean the tracheostomy site

D) Leave the tracheostomy site uncovered to allow for ventilation

46. What is the purpose of using a splint?

A) To immobilize and support an injured limb or joint

B) To enhance the range of motion in a joint

C) To provide comfort during mobility exercises

D) To treat infections in the affected area

47. How should a CNA assist a patient with a mobility aid?

A) Ensure the aid is properly fitted and the patient is comfortable using it

B) Remove the mobility aid if the patient prefers to walk without assistance

C) Use the mobility aid only if the patient requests it

D) Allow the patient to use the aid independently without supervision

48. When performing passive range-of-motion exercises, what is important?

A) Move the joints gently and within the patient's comfort level

B) Apply force to stretch the muscles and increase flexibility

C) Perform the exercises quickly to save time

D) Limit the range of motion to avoid causing pain

49. How should a CNA assist a patient with a colostomy?

A) Monitor the stoma for changes and empty the bag as needed

B) Remove the colostomy bag and leave the stoma uncovered for ventilation

C) Use non-sterile wipes to clean the stoma

D) Restrict the patient's diet to prevent leakage

50. What is the appropriate method for handling a patient's personal belongings?

A) Keep belongings organized and within reach of the patient

B) Store belongings in a common area for safety

C) Discard any items that are not immediately needed

D) Allow only authorized personnel to handle personal items

51. How should a CNA manage a patient with a feeding tube?

A) Verify tube placement and ensure proper feeding technique

B) Administer feedings while the patient is lying flat

C) Use a non-sterile technique to clean the feeding tube

D) Avoid flushing the tube to prevent blockages

52. What is the correct procedure for measuring a patient's blood glucose level?

A) Cleanse the patient's finger, use a lancet, and apply blood to a test strip

B) Use a continuous glucose monitor without obtaining a fingerstick sample

C) Measure glucose levels through a urine sample

D) Collect a blood sample from the patient's arm

53. When assisting a patient with ambulation, what is an essential consideration?

A) Use proper body mechanics and provide support as needed

B) Encourage the patient to walk without any assistance

C) Restrict the patient's movement to prevent falls

D) Allow the patient to walk independently without supervision

54. What is the purpose of applying a warm compress?

A) To promote circulation and alleviate pain

B) To cool down a fever and reduce body temperature

C) To cleanse wounds and prevent infection

D) To numb the area and reduce sensitivity

55. How should a CNA handle a patient with impaired vision?

A) Describe the environment and provide assistance with navigation

B) Avoid making any modifications to the environment

C) Allow the patient to navigate independently without assistance

D) Use bright lights to enhance visibility

56. What is the proper method for collecting a urine sample?

Use a sterile container and collect the sample mid-stream

Collect the sample from the patient's bedside commode

Use a non-sterile container and obtain the sample after the patient has finished

Collect the sample directly from the catheter bag

57. When assisting with a patient's bath, what is important?

A) Ensure privacy and provide a comfortable, warm environment

B) Use hot water to clean the patient quickly

C) Avoid using soap to prevent skin irritation

D) Perform the bath as quickly as possible

58. What should a CNA do if a patient has difficulty swallowing?

A) Modify the patient's diet to include soft or pureed foods and report the issue

B) Encourage the patient to eat solid foods and drink fluids quickly

C) Avoid modifying the diet and allow the patient to eat independently

D) Administer thickening agents without consulting a nurse

59. What is the purpose of performing a skin assessment?

A) To detect and address changes in skin condition and prevent complications

B) To assess the patient's overall health and well-being

C) To ensure the patient is comfortable and free of discomfort

D) To evaluate the effectiveness of wound healing

60. How should a CNA assist a patient with a cast?

A) Elevate the casted limb and monitor for signs of swelling

B) Remove the cast if the patient reports discomfort

C) Allow the cast to become wet during bathing

D) Apply pressure to the cast to ensure proper fitting

61. What is the correct procedure for administering a subcutaneous injection?

A) Cleanse the skin with alcohol, insert the needle at a 45-degree angle, and inject the medication

B) Insert the needle directly into the muscle and inject the medication

C) Use a large gauge needle and inject the medication quickly

D) Avoid using alcohol swabs and inject the medication without aspiration

62. How should a CNA handle a patient with a feeding tube?

A) Verify tube placement and flush with water before and after feeding

B) Leave the tube disconnected to allow for air circulation

C) Feed the patient while they are lying flat in bed

D) Avoid using sterile equipment during the feeding process

63. What is the purpose of using an incentive spirometer?

A) To encourage deep breathing and prevent lung complications

B) To measure oxygen saturation levels in the blood

C) To assess respiratory rate and rhythm

D) To provide supplemental oxygen to the patient

64. When performing wound care, what is a key step?

A) Clean the wound with an appropriate solution and apply a sterile dressing

B) Apply ointment without cleaning the wound first

C) Leave the wound uncovered to promote air healing

D) Use non-sterile gloves to handle the wound

65. How should a CNA manage a patient with a tracheostomy?

A) Ensure the tracheostomy tube is clear and clean the area around it

B) Remove the tracheostomy tube if the patient is uncomfortable

C) Avoid monitoring the tracheostomy site unless the patient complains

D) Use non-sterile wipes to clean the tracheostomy site

66. What is the proper technique for measuring a patient's weight?

A) Use a calibrated scale and have the patient stand still for an accurate reading

B) Weigh the patient while seated in a chair or wheelchair

C) Estimate the patient's weight based on their body size

D) Measure weight without removing any clothing or accessories

67. How should a CNA assist a patient with a walker?

A) Ensure the walker is adjusted to the correct height and provide support during movement

B) Push the walker for the patient to assist with walking

C) Allow the patient to use the walker independently without assistance

D) Remove the walker if the patient is comfortable walking without it

68. What is the purpose of performing passive range-of-motion exercises?

A) To maintain joint flexibility and prevent stiffness

B) To increase muscle strength and endurance

C) To improve cardiovascular fitness

D) To promote relaxation and reduce stress

69. How should a CNA handle a patient with an intravenous (IV) line?

A) Monitor the IV site for signs of infection and ensure proper flow

B) Change the IV site without consulting a nurse

C) Administer medications through the IV line without authorization

D) Remove the IV line if the patient experiences discomfort

70. What is the correct way to perform oral care for a patient with dentures?

A) Clean the dentures with a denture brush and place them in a denture cup

B) Brush the dentures with regular toothpaste and leave them in the patient's mouth

C) Clean the dentures with water only and store them in a drawer

D) Remove the dentures and leave them out of the patient's mouth

71. When assisting with an enema, what should a CNA do?

A) Ensure the patient is in a comfortable position and follow proper hygiene practices

B) Use a non-sterile enema kit and administer the enema quickly

C) Perform the procedure without asking the patient's consent

D) Remove the enema if the patient experiences discomfort

72. What is the appropriate method for performing catheter care?

A) Cleanse the catheter and surrounding area with sterile water and avoid pulling on the catheter

B) Use non-sterile wipes to clean the catheter and change it daily

C) Remove the catheter if the patient shows signs of discomfort

D) Allow the catheter to remain in place without any cleaning

73. How should a CNA manage a patient who is at risk for pressure ulcers?

A) Reposition the patient frequently and use pressure-relieving devices

B) Restrict the patient's mobility to prevent pressure sores

C) Use only a standard mattress without additional cushioning

D) Avoid inspecting the skin to prevent disturbing the patient

74. What is the correct procedure for measuring blood pressure?

A) Place the cuff around the patient's upper arm and inflate it to measure systolic and diastolic pressures

B) Measure blood pressure on the patient's wrist and use a digital monitor

C) Inflate the cuff until it is tight and then slowly release the pressure

D) Measure blood pressure on the patient's thigh and record the reading

75. When assisting a patient with a wheelchair, what is important?

A) Ensure the wheelchair is locked before assisting with transfers

B) Allow the patient to push the wheelchair independently without assistance

C) Remove the footrests and armrests to facilitate easier transfers

D) Leave the wheelchair unlocked to allow for easy movement

76. What is the purpose of using a nasal cannula?

A) To provide supplemental oxygen to patients with respiratory issues

B) To administer medication directly into the nasal passages

C) To measure oxygen saturation levels in the blood

D) To assess the patient's respiratory rate and rhythm

77. How should a CNA handle a patient with a splint?

A) Elevate the splinted limb and monitor for any signs of swelling or discomfort

B) Remove the splint if the patient reports pain or discomfort

C) Allow the splint to become wet during bathing

D) Apply pressure to the splint to ensure a snug fit

78. What is the correct technique for performing passive range-of-motion exercises?

A) Move each joint through its full range of motion gently and slowly

B) Stretch each joint aggressively to increase flexibility

C) Perform the exercises quickly to save time

D) Limit movement to avoid causing pain

79. When assisting with a patient's personal hygiene, what should a CNA do?

A) Ensure privacy, use appropriate hygiene products, and respect the patient's preferences

B) Rush through the process to complete it quickly

C) Use only one type of hygiene product for all tasks

D) Perform the hygiene tasks without consulting the patient

80. How should a CNA handle a patient who is exhibiting signs of agitation?

A) Remain calm, offer reassurance, and report the behavior to the nurse

B) Avoid any interaction to prevent further agitation

C) Restrict the patient's movement to control their behavior

D) Administer medication to calm the patient without authorization

81. What is the correct method for measuring an infant's head circumference?

A) Use a flexible measuring tape and measure around the widest part of the head
B) Measure the head circumference while the infant is lying flat in bed
C) Use a rigid ruler and measure from the forehead to the back of the head
D) Estimate the head circumference based on the infant's age

82. How should a CNA assist a patient with a colostomy bag?

A) Monitor the bag for leaks, empty it as needed, and keep the area clean
B) Remove the colostomy bag if the patient reports discomfort
C) Use non-sterile wipes to clean the stoma
D) Restrict the patient's diet to prevent leakage

83. What is the purpose of using an air mattress for a patient?

A) To reduce the risk of pressure ulcers by providing even pressure distribution
B) To increase the patient's comfort during sleep
C) To support the patient's back and improve posture
D) To warm the patient's body during cold weather

84. When performing a skin assessment, what should a CNA look for?

A) Changes in skin color, temperature, and texture
B) The patient's overall mood and emotional state
C) The patient's recent dietary intake
D) The patient's mobility and activity level

85. How should a CNA handle a patient with a nasogastric (NG) tube?

A) Verify tube placement before feeding and flush the tube as needed

B) Avoid checking the tube placement and feed the patient without verification

C) Administer feedings while the patient is lying flat in bed

D) Use non-sterile techniques to handle the NG tube

86. What is the correct procedure for measuring a patient's respiratory rate?

A) Observe the patient's chest rise and fall for one minute

B) Count the number of breaths for 30 seconds and multiply by 2

C) Measure the respiratory rate while the patient is talking

D) Use a stethoscope to listen to the patient's lungs for 5 minutes

87. How should a CNA manage a patient with a chronic illness?

A) Provide regular monitoring and care as directed by the healthcare provider

B) Focus only on the patient's immediate needs and ignore long-term management

C) Allow the patient to manage their condition independently without assistance

D) Restrict the patient's activities to prevent complications

88. What is the purpose of a foot care routine for diabetic patients?

A) To prevent infections and complications related to poor circulation

B) To enhance the appearance of the feet and toenails

C) To provide comfort and relaxation to the feet

D) To assess the patient's overall health status

89. How should a CNA assist a patient with a chest tube?

A) Monitor the chest tube for proper drainage and ensure it is securely attached

B) Remove the chest tube if the patient experiences discomfort

C) Allow the chest tube to become disconnected during movement

D) Clean the chest tube with non-sterile wipes

90. What is the correct procedure for measuring a patient's pulse?

A) Place fingers over the patient's radial artery and count beats for one minute

B) Use a pulse oximeter to measure the pulse rate

C) Measure the pulse rate by listening to the heart with a stethoscope

D) Count the number of beats for 30 seconds and multiply by 4

91. How should a CNA manage a patient with dementia?

A) Use simple, clear communication and provide a structured routine

B) Avoid interacting with the patient to prevent confusion

C) Change the patient's routine frequently to stimulate mental activity

D) Restrict the patient's activities to prevent agitation

92. What is the purpose of a pressure-relieving cushion?

A) To reduce pressure on the skin and prevent pressure ulcers

B) To enhance the patient's comfort during sitting

C) To improve posture and alignment

D) To support the patient's lower back

93. How should a CNA handle a patient who is refusing medication?

A) Respect the patient's decision and report the refusal to the nurse

B) Force the medication into the patient's mouth to ensure compliance

C) Ignore the refusal and administer the medication later

D) Administer the medication without the patient's consent

94. What is the appropriate method for collecting a stool sample?

A) Use a sterile container and collect the sample from a fresh bowel movement

B) Collect the sample from the patient's bedpan and store it for later use

C) Use a non-sterile container and obtain the sample from the toilet bowl

D) Collect the sample directly from the catheter bag

95. How should a CNA assist a patient with mobility issues?

A) Provide support and use assistive devices as needed for safe movement

B) Encourage the patient to move independently without assistance

C) Restrict the patient's movement to prevent falls

D) Remove assistive devices to encourage physical activity

96. What is the purpose of using a bedpan or urinal?

A) To provide a convenient method for patients to relieve themselves when immobile

B) To assist patients with maintaining personal hygiene

C) To monitor urine output for medical evaluation

D) To prevent patients from getting out of bed

97. How should a CNA handle a patient with a seizure?

A) Protect the patient from injury, place them on their side, and seek medical assistance

B) Hold the patient down to prevent excessive movement

C) Restrict the patient's movement to stop the seizure

D) Administer anti-seizure medication without consulting a nurse

98. What is the correct procedure for measuring a patient's temperature?

A) Use a thermometer and place it under the patient's tongue, in their armpit, or rectally as indicated

B) Measure temperature using a non-contact infrared thermometer on the patient's forehead

C) Take temperature readings by placing a thermometer in the patient's ear

D) Estimate the temperature based on the patient's overall condition

99. How should a CNA assist a patient with speech difficulties?

A) Use simple, clear language and allow extra time for the patient to respond

B) Speak for the patient to expedite communication

C) Ignore the patient's attempts to speak if they are struggling

D) Avoid any conversation to prevent frustration

100. What is the purpose of using a transfer belt?

A) To assist with safe patient transfers and provide support during movement

B) To restrict the patient's movement and prevent falls

C) To monitor the patient's vital signs during transfers

D) To measure the patient's waist size for clothing adjustment

ANSWERS

1. A:	21. A:.	41. D:	61. A:	81. A
2. A:	22. A.	42. A:	62. A	82. A
3. A:	23. A	43. A.	63. A	83. A:
4. A:	24. A:	44. A.	64. A	84. A:
5. A:	25. A:	45. A	65. A:	85. A:.
6. A:	26. A	46. A	66. A:	86. A
7. A:	27. A:	47. A:	67. A:.	87. A
8. A	28. A	48. A	68. A	88. A
9. A:.	29. A:	49. A	69. A	89. A:
10. A	30. A	50. A	70. A:	90. A
11. A:.	31. A.	51. A	71. A	91. A:
12. A:.	32. A.	52. A:	72. A	92. A:.
13. A.	33. A.	53. A	73. A:	93. A:.
14. A.	34. A	54. A:	74. A:	94. A
15. A:	35. A	55. A:.	75. A	95. A
16. A.	36. A:	56. A	76. A	96. A:
17. A:.	37. A:	57. A	77. A	97. A:
18. A.	38. A	58. A	78. A.	98. A
19. A:.	39. A:	59. A:	79. A	99. A:
20. A:	40. A:	60. A	80. A:	100. A

CHAPTER THREE
QUESTION AND ANSWERS

1. **What is the primary purpose of effective communication in patient care?**

    A) To complete documentation quickly

    B) To build a rapport and ensure understanding between patient and caregiver

    C) To meet institutional regulations

    D) To manage multiple patients at once

2. **How should a CNA respond to a patient who is anxious about an upcoming procedure?**

    A) Ignore their anxiety and proceed with the procedure

    B) Reassure the patient and provide clear information about the procedure

    C) Avoid discussing the procedure to prevent further anxiety

    D) Rush through the procedure to minimize their worry

3. **What is an appropriate way to handle a patient's complaint about pain?**

    A) Dismiss the complaint as a minor issue

    B) Report the complaint to the nurse and document it accurately

    C) Provide pain medication without authorization

    D) Advise the patient to endure the pain as part of their recovery

4. **How should a CNA communicate with a patient who is hard of hearing?**

    A) Speak loudly and slowly, and use gestures or written notes

B) Avoid talking and use non-verbal cues only

C) Speak normally and assume the patient can understand

D) Shout to get their attention

5 What is the best way to maintain patient privacy during a conversation?

A) Discuss patient information in public areas where others may overhear

B) Ensure conversations are held in private settings and use discretion

C) Use vague language to avoid disclosing specific details

D) Only discuss patient information when absolutely necessary

6 How can a CNA support a patient who is feeling depressed?

A) Offer distractions and try to cheer them up with jokes

B) Listen empathetically and provide a supportive presence

C) Tell them to focus on positive aspects of their situation

D) Suggest they see a mental health specialist without consulting their healthcare provider

7 What is the role of active listening in patient care?

A) To complete tasks more efficiently

B) To ensure the patient's needs and concerns are fully understood and addressed

C) To avoid unnecessary conversations with the patient

D) To follow institutional communication protocols

8 How should a CNA handle a situation where a patient is refusing to eat?

A) Force the patient to eat to ensure they receive proper nutrition

B) Ignore the refusal and document the patient's intake

C) Discuss the reasons for refusal with the patient and report to the nurse

D) Provide alternative foods without discussing the refusal

9 When should a CNA report changes in a patient's condition to the nurse?

A) Only when asked about the changes

B) At the end of their shift to avoid interruptions

C) Immediately when noticed to ensure timely intervention

D) Only if the changes seem severe

10 What is an appropriate action if a patient is displaying aggressive behavior?

A) Confront the patient aggressively to assert control

B) Remain calm, use non-threatening body language, and seek help if needed

C) Avoid the patient and report the behavior at the end of the shift

D) Restrict the patient's movement to prevent further aggression

11 How should a CNA address a patient who is confused about their surroundings?

A) Ignore their confusion and proceed with the task at hand

B) Provide reassurance, orient the patient to their surroundings, and offer assistance

C) Tell the patient that they need to remember their surroundings better

D) Provide a detailed explanation of their surroundings in a complicated manner

12 **What is the best way to communicate with a patient who is unable to speak?**

   A) Speak directly to the patient and wait for a response

   B) Speak to the patient's family members instead

   C) Assume the patient does not understand and provide information to others

   D) Use alternative communication methods, such as writing or communication boards

13 **How should a CNA handle a patient's cultural or religious preferences during care?**

   A) Ignore the preferences and follow standard procedures

   B) Respect the preferences and incorporate them into the care plan where possible

   C) Discuss the preferences with the patient only if they bring it up

   D) Modify the care plan to meet the preferences only if it is convenient

14 **What is the appropriate response if a patient expresses fear about a diagnosis?**

   A) Minimize their concerns and change the subject

   B) Listen to their fears, provide supportive reassurance, and involve the healthcare team

   C) Tell them to accept the diagnosis and move on

   D) Avoid discussing the diagnosis further

15 **How should a CNA handle a situation where a patient has fallen out of bed?**

A) Immediately lift the patient back into bed without assessing for injuries

B) Assess the patient for injuries, call for help, and then move the patient if necessary

C) Ignore the fall if the patient appears to be fine

D) Only document the fall and inform the nurse later

16 What is the best way to communicate with a patient who is anxious about their treatment?

A) Provide clear, concise information about the treatment and offer reassurance

B) Avoid discussing the treatment to prevent further anxiety

C) Rush through the explanation to get it over with

D) Tell the patient not to worry and proceed with the treatment

17 How can a CNA promote patient dignity during personal care?

A) Provide care efficiently but without considering the patient's comfort

B) Maintain the patient's privacy, use respectful language, and involve them in decisions

C) Discuss the care process with others to ensure accuracy

D) Perform tasks quickly to minimize the patient's embarrassment

18 What should a CNA do if a patient expresses dissatisfaction with their care?

A) Ignore the complaint and continue with the care

B) Listen to the patient's concerns, address them appropriately, and report to the nurse

C) Tell the patient that their complaints are not valid

D) Document the dissatisfaction and report it at the end of the shift

19 How should a CNA handle a situation where a patient is unable to communicate verbally?

A) Assume the patient does not need any assistance

B) Use alternative communication methods such as gestures, writing, or communication aids

C) Avoid interacting with the patient and wait for them to communicate

D) Only speak to family members or caregivers about the patient's needs

20 What is the best way to ensure effective handoff communication between shifts?

A) Quickly relay only the most critical information to the next shift

B) Provide a detailed and organized report including patient status, needs, and any concerns

C) Discuss patient care informally with the next shift without documentation

D) Assume that the next shift is aware of all the details from the previous shift

21 How should a CNA respond if a patient requests information about their medical condition?

A) Provide detailed medical explanations as per the CNA's knowledge

B) Direct the patient to speak with their healthcare provider or nurse for detailed information

C) Avoid discussing the condition to prevent misinformation

D) Give general information without ensuring accuracy

22 What is the appropriate way to assist a patient who is in a wheelchair and needs to be transferred to a bed?

　　A) Move the patient without using any assistive devices or techniques
　　B) Use proper body mechanics, and ensure the wheelchair is locked before transferring
　　C) Ask the patient to move themselves with minimal assistance
　　D) Perform the transfer quickly to reduce discomfort

23 How should a CNA deal with a patient who refuses to follow care instructions?

　　A) Force the patient to comply with the instructions
　　B) Discuss the reasons for refusal with the patient, and inform the healthcare team
　　C) Ignore the refusal and proceed with care as usual
　　D) Change the care instructions without consulting the healthcare team

24 What is the best approach to take when providing care for a patient with limited mobility?

　　A) Allow the patient to move independently and only assist when absolutely necessary
　　B) Use assistive devices and support the patient in moving safely and comfortably
　　C) Restrict the patient's movement to prevent accidents
　　D) Perform all tasks for the patient to minimize their physical effort

25 **How should a CNA handle a situation where a patient expresses feelings of loneliness?**

   A) Ignore their feelings and continue with care tasks
   B) Spend time with the patient, offer companionship, and involve them in activities
   C) Encourage the patient to focus on their treatment to forget their loneliness
   D) Suggest they contact family members or friends on their own

26 **What is the most appropriate action if a patient is experiencing difficulty breathing?**

   A) Provide supplemental oxygen without authorization
   B) Position the patient in an upright position and call for immediate medical assistance
   C) Avoid disturbing the patient and wait to see if the issue resolves

D) Administer medication if the patient has a prescription for it

27 **How should a CNA address a patient who is showing signs of delirium?**

   A) Ignore the symptoms and continue with routine care
   B) Ensure the patient's safety, provide a calm environment, and notify the healthcare team
   C) Restrict the patient's movement to prevent injury
   D) Confront the patient about their confusion and try to correct it

28 **What is the best way to communicate with a patient who has limited English proficiency?**

A) Speak slowly and loudly, using simple words

B) Use a translator or interpreter to ensure clear communication

C) Rely on gestures and body language to communicate

D) Avoid discussing complex topics and only provide basic information

29 **How should a CNA approach a patient who is refusing to take medication?**

A) Force the medication on the patient to ensure they receive their treatment

B) Explain the importance of the medication, discuss any concerns, and report to the nurse

C) Ignore the refusal and document the medication as given

D) Provide the medication at a later time without addressing the refusal

30 **What is an effective strategy for a CNA to use when dealing with a non-compliant patient?**

A) Force compliance through authoritative measures

B) Engage the patient in discussion, understand their reasons for non-compliance, and involve them in their care plan

C) Avoid interacting with the patient to prevent conflict

D) Document the non-compliance and report it without further action

31 **What is the best approach to take when managing a patient's pain?**

A) Administer pain relief medication as frequently as possible

B) Assess the patient's pain level, provide comfort measures, and report to the nurse for further intervention

C) Ignore the pain if it seems manageable

D) Ask the patient to wait until the next scheduled medication time

32 How should a CNA respond if a patient is upset about the care they are receiving?

   A) Defend the care provided and explain why it was necessary
   B) Listen to the patient's concerns, apologize for any issues, and work to resolve them
   C) Ignore the complaint and continue with care as usual
   D) Suggest the patient speak with the nurse to resolve their issues

33 What is the best way to ensure patient safety during a transfer?

   A) Perform the transfer quickly to minimize the time the patient is at risk
   B) Use proper body mechanics, provide support, and ensure the patient is securely positioned
   C) Allow the patient to assist as much as possible without providing support
   D) Complete the transfer without any additional equipment or assistance

34 How should a CNA handle a situation where a patient's family is demanding information about the patient's condition?

   A) Provide detailed information to the family without considering patient privacy
   B) Share information only with the patient's consent or direct the family to speak with the healthcare team
   C) Avoid discussing the patient's condition with the family altogether
   D) Give general information but avoid specifics about the patient's health

35 What is an appropriate response when a patient exhibits signs of dehydration?

   A) Increase the patient's fluid intake and document the signs of dehydration
   B) Ignore the signs and monitor the patient for changes
   C) Administer intravenous fluids without authorization
   D) Advise the patient to drink more fluids and wait for improvement

36 How can a CNA best support a patient who is going through a difficult emotional time?

   A) Distract the patient with entertainment or activities
   B) Provide a listening ear, offer emotional support, and involve the healthcare team if needed
   C) Suggest the patient focus on positive thoughts and avoid discussing their emotions
   D) Leave the patient alone to process their emotions independently

37 What is the best way to communicate with a patient who is disoriented?

   A) Speak clearly and slowly, use simple language, and provide reassurance
   B) Avoid talking to the patient until they are more alert
   C) Provide detailed explanations about their condition and surroundings
   D) Speak to the patient's family members for more effective communication

38 How should a CNA handle a situation where a patient is exhibiting symptoms of an allergic reaction?

   A) Ignore the symptoms and monitor the patient for changes

B) Report the symptoms to the nurse immediately and provide first aid if trained to do so

C) Administer an antihistamine without authorization

D) Document the symptoms and wait for the healthcare team to address them

39 What is the best approach to take when a patient is expressing frustration about their treatment plan?

A) Ignore the patient's frustration and continue with the treatment plan

B) Discuss the patient's concerns, provide explanations, and collaborate on adjustments to the plan if appropriate

C) Tell the patient to follow the plan without question

D) Redirect the conversation to avoid discussing the treatment plan

40 How should a CNA respond if a patient is experiencing nausea?

A) Provide the patient with a variety of foods to choose from

B) Offer small sips of clear fluids, report the symptom to the nurse, and document it

C) Ignore the nausea and continue with other care tasks

D) Administer anti-nausea medication without authorization

41 What is an effective way for a CNA to assist a patient with activities of daily living (ADLs)?

A) Perform all tasks for the patient to ensure they are done correctly

B) Encourage the patient to perform as many ADLs as they can independently, providing assistance as needed

C) Limit the patient's involvement to prevent them from exerting too much effort

D) Only assist with ADLs if the patient specifically requests help

42 How should a CNA handle a situation where a patient is having difficulty swallowing?

A) Offer the patient foods that are easy to swallow without addressing the difficulty

B) Report the swallowing difficulty to the nurse, and modify the patient's diet as advised

C) Ignore the issue and continue with feeding as usual

D) Administer thickening agents without authorization

43 What is the best way to support a patient who is undergoing physical therapy?

A) Provide encouragement and assist with exercises as directed by the therapist

B) Allow the patient to complete exercises independently without any support

C) Avoid participating in the therapy process to prevent interfering

D) Perform the exercises for the patient to ensure they are done correctly

44 How should a CNA approach a patient who is experiencing difficulty with mobility?

A) Encourage the patient to walk as much as possible, even if it causes discomfort

B) Assist the patient with mobility aids, and provide support and encouragement while ensuring safety

C) Restrict the patient's mobility to prevent falls

D) Allow the patient to remain in bed to avoid any mobility issues

45 What is the best approach to take when communicating with a patient who has cognitive impairments?

A) Use complex sentences and medical terminology to provide detailed explanations

B) Speak clearly, use simple language, and offer visual aids if needed

C) Assume the patient cannot understand and avoid engaging in conversation

D) Provide information only to the patient's family members

46 How should a CNA handle a situation where a patient is refusing to follow hygiene practices?

A) Force the patient to follow hygiene practices for their health

B) Discuss the importance of hygiene, address any concerns, and provide assistance as needed

C) Ignore the refusal and document it as non-compliance

D) Modify hygiene practices without consulting the patient or healthcare team

47 What is the best way to provide end-of-life care to a patient?

A) Focus on the patient's physical needs and ignore emotional and spiritual support

B) Provide comfort measures, listen to the patient's needs, and involve the patient's family and support systems

C) Continue with aggressive treatments to prolong life

D) Minimize contact with the patient to avoid emotional distress

48 How should a CNA respond if a patient is experiencing pain during a procedure?

   A) Continue with the procedure and advise the patient to endure the pain
   B) Stop the procedure, assess the patient's pain level, and notify the nurse for further instructions
   C) Ignore the patient's pain and proceed as planned
   D) Provide pain relief medication without authorization

49 What is the best way to manage a patient's dietary restrictions?

   A) Ignore the restrictions and provide the patient with standard meals
   B) Follow the dietary restrictions carefully, and coordinate with the dietary department to ensure compliance
   C) Provide alternative foods without considering the restrictions
   D) Discuss the restrictions with the patient only if they ask

50 How should a CNA handle a situation where a patient is upset about their living conditions?

   A) Dismiss their concerns and continue with care tasks
   B) Listen to the patient's concerns, address them respectfully, and report any issues to the appropriate personnel
   C) Avoid discussing the living conditions and focus on other aspects of care
   D) Suggest the patient speak with management about their concerns

51 What is the best approach for a CNA to take when dealing with a patient's challenging behavior?

   A) Confront the patient about their behavior aggressively

B) Remain calm, use de-escalation techniques, and seek support from the healthcare team

C) Ignore the behavior and continue with care as usual

D) Restrict the patient's privileges to correct the behavior

52 **How should a CNA respond if a patient asks about their treatment options?**

A) Provide detailed medical explanations and discuss options in depth

B) Direct the patient to their healthcare provider or nurse for information about treatment options

C) Offer general information without specifics to avoid misinformation

D) Avoid discussing treatment options to prevent confusion

53 **What is the appropriate action if a patient has a new or worsening symptom?**

A) Document the symptom and wait for the next scheduled assessment

B) Report the new or worsening symptom to the nurse immediately for further evaluation

C) Ignore the symptom if it seems minor

D) Treat the symptom with over-the-counter medication if appropriate

54 **How should a CNA assist a patient with their personal hygiene needs?**

A) Complete all hygiene tasks for the patient without involving them

B) Provide assistance as needed, respecting the patient's preferences and promoting independence

C) Perform hygiene tasks quickly to minimize discomfort

D) Only assist with hygiene if the patient explicitly requests help

55 What is the best way to communicate with a patient who is in severe pain?

A) Minimize communication and focus on pain relief measures

B) Speak calmly, provide reassurance, and involve the healthcare team to address the pain effectively

C) Avoid discussing the pain to prevent further distress

D) Provide pain relief medication without authorization

56 How should a CNA approach a patient who is anxious about an upcoming surgery?

A) Reassure the patient with general statements and avoid detailed information
B) Provide clear, accurate information about the procedure and offer emotional support
C) Ignore the patient's anxiety and focus on preparing them for the surgery
D) Advise the patient to remain calm and not worry about the surgery

57 What is the best way to handle a situation where a patient has difficulty understanding instructions?

A) Repeat the instructions in a complex manner for clarity
B) Use simple, clear language, and provide visual aids or demonstrations if needed

C) Avoid providing instructions and assume the patient will understand eventually

D) Provide written instructions without offering verbal explanations

58 **How should a CNA respond if a patient is exhibiting signs of emotional distress?**

A) Ignore the distress and continue with care tasks

B) Offer a supportive presence, listen to the patient's concerns, and involve the healthcare team if needed

C) Encourage the patient to focus on positive aspects and avoid discussing their distress

D) Advise the patient to seek help from family or friends

59 **What is an appropriate response if a patient expresses dissatisfaction with their care plan?**

A) Ignore the patient's dissatisfaction and continue with the care plan

B) Discuss the patient's concerns, provide explanations, and collaborate on possible adjustments to the care plan

C) Tell the patient that their dissatisfaction is not valid

D) Redirect the conversation to avoid discussing the care plan

60 **How should a CNA address a patient's concern about a change in their medication regimen?**

A) Provide detailed explanations about the medication change

B) Direct the patient to speak with their healthcare provider or pharmacist for detailed information

C) Ignore the concern and continue with the new medication regimen

D) Offer general information about medication changes without specifics

61 What is the best approach to take when working with a patient who has a cognitive impairment?

A) Use complex instructions to ensure the patient understands the care plan

B) Provide simple, clear instructions, and use repetitive reminders if necessary

C) Assume the patient cannot understand and avoid discussing their care needs

D) Only involve the patient's family members in the care process

62 How should a CNA handle a situation where a patient is feeling isolated due to a long hospital stay?

A) Ignore the patient's feelings and focus on medical care

B) Provide companionship, engage in conversations, and involve the patient in social activities if possible

C) Encourage the patient to focus on their recovery and avoid discussing their isolation

D) Suggest the patient contact family or friends to alleviate their feelings of isolation

63 What is the best way to assist a patient who is experiencing difficulty with self-care tasks?

A) Perform all tasks for the patient without considering their input

B) Offer assistance as needed, encourage independence, and provide support for self-care tasks

C) Limit the patient's involvement in self-care to prevent mistakes

D) Only assist if the patient specifically requests help

64 **How should a CNA approach a patient who is experiencing difficulty with mobility?**

A) Encourage the patient to walk independently without any assistance
B) Provide support and use mobility aids as needed to ensure safety during movement
C) Restrict the patient's movement to prevent falls and injuries
D) Perform all mobility tasks for the patient to avoid any risk

65 **What is the best way to communicate with a patient who has limited cognitive function?**

A) Use complex sentences and medical terminology for detailed explanations
B) Speak slowly, use simple language, and provide visual aids or demonstrations if necessary
C) Assume the patient cannot understand and avoid engaging in conversation
D) Provide information only to the patient's family members

66 **How should a CNA handle a situation where a patient is refusing to participate in physical therapy?**

A) Force the patient to participate in therapy to ensure they follow the plan
B) Discuss the reasons for refusal with the patient, address any concerns, and report to the healthcare team
C) Ignore the refusal and proceed with other care tasks
D) Modify the therapy plan without consulting the patient or healthcare team

67 **What is the best way to provide care for a patient with a chronic illness?**

A) Focus solely on managing the illness without considering the patient's overall well-being

B) Provide comprehensive care that addresses both the chronic illness and the patient's overall comfort and needs

C) Limit care to only addressing symptoms of the chronic illness

D) Provide care as per the standard protocol without individualizing it

68 How should a CNA address a patient's concerns about a new treatment plan?

A) Provide detailed medical explanations and address all concerns

B) Direct the patient to speak with their healthcare provider for detailed information about the treatment plan

C) Avoid discussing the new treatment plan to prevent confusion

D) Offer general information about the treatment plan without specifics

69 What is the best approach for a CNA to take when dealing with a patient's fear of a medical procedure?

A) Reassure the patient with vague statements and proceed with the procedure

B) Provide clear, accurate information about the procedure, address their fears, and offer emotional support

C) Avoid discussing the procedure to prevent further anxiety

D) Rush through the procedure to minimize the patient's fear

70 How should a CNA respond if a patient is experiencing discomfort during a procedure?

A) Continue with the procedure and advise the patient to endure the discomfort

B) Stop the procedure, assess the patient's comfort level, and notify the nurse for further instructions

C) Ignore the discomfort and proceed as planned

D) Provide discomfort relief measures without authorization

71 **What is the best way to communicate with a patient who is feeling overwhelmed by their diagnosis?**

A) Offer general reassurance without discussing the diagnosis in detail

B) Provide empathetic support, offer information about the diagnosis, and involve the healthcare team for additional support

C) Avoid discussing the diagnosis to prevent overwhelming the patient

D) Suggest the patient focus on treatment to distract from their diagnosis

72 **How should a CNA approach a patient who is experiencing difficulty breathing?**

A) Ignore the difficulty and continue with other care tasks

B) Position the patient in a comfortable position, monitor their breathing, and seek immediate medical assistance if necessary

C) Provide supplemental oxygen without authorization

D) Encourage the patient to breathe deeply and wait for improvement

73 **What is the best way to handle a situation where a patient is refusing to take their prescribed medications?**

A) Force the patient to take the medications to ensure adherence

B) Discuss the reasons for refusal with the patient, provide education on the importance of the medications, and report to the healthcare team

C) Ignore the refusal and document it as non-compliance

D) Administer the medications at a later time without addressing the refusal

74 How should a CNA address a patient's concerns about their dietary needs?

A) Provide the patient with standard meals without considering their dietary needs

B) Address the patient's concerns, follow their dietary preferences, and coordinate with the dietary department to ensure compliance

C) Ignore the dietary needs and focus on other aspects of care

D) Offer general food options without regard to the patient's dietary restrictions

75 What is the best way to support a patient who is feeling isolated due to their condition?

A) Ignore the patient's feelings and continue with medical care

B) Provide emotional support, engage in conversation, and involve the patient in social activities if possible

C) Encourage the patient to focus on their condition to distract from their feelings of isolation

D) Suggest the patient contact family or friends for support

76 How should a CNA respond if a patient is experiencing symptoms of infection?

A) Ignore the symptoms and continue with other care tasks

B) Report the symptoms to the nurse immediately, and follow infection control protocols

C) Administer antibiotics without authorization

D) Provide comfort measures and document the symptoms for later review

77 What is the appropriate action if a patient expresses frustration with their care team?

A) Defend the care team and explain their actions

B) Listen to the patient's concerns, acknowledge their feelings, and work with the care team to address the issues

C) Ignore the frustration and continue with care as usual

D) Suggest the patient speak with management about their concerns

78 How should a CNA approach a patient who is feeling anxious about their treatment plan?

A) Provide general reassurance without discussing specifics about the treatment plan

B) Offer clear, accurate information about the treatment plan, address their concerns, and provide emotional support

C) Avoid discussing the treatment plan to prevent further anxiety

D) Rush through the discussion to minimize the patient's anxiety

79 What is the best way to handle a situation where a patient is refusing to participate in a care plan?

A) Force the patient to participate to ensure adherence to the care plan

B) Discuss the reasons for refusal with the patient, address their concerns, and report to the healthcare team for further action

C) Ignore the refusal and proceed with other care tasks

D) Modify the care plan without consulting the patient or healthcare team

80   How should a CNA assist a patient who is experiencing difficulty with their breathing?

A) Ignore the breathing difficulty and continue with other care tasks

B) Position the patient in a comfortable position, monitor their breathing, and seek medical assistance if necessary

C) Provide supplemental oxygen without authorization

D) Encourage the patient to breathe deeply and wait for improvement

81   What is the best way to provide care to a patient who is struggling with a chronic condition?

A) Focus only on managing symptoms without addressing the patient's overall well-being

B) Provide comprehensive care that considers both the chronic condition and the patient's overall comfort and needs

C) Limit care to only addressing the chronic condition's symptoms

D) Follow standard care protocols without considering the patient's individual needs

82   How should a CNA handle a situation where a patient is experiencing confusion or disorientation?

A) Provide detailed explanations about their condition and surroundings

B) Speak clearly and calmly, use simple language, and offer reassurance

C) Avoid interacting with the patient to prevent further confusion

D) Speak to the patient's family members for better communication

83   What is the best approach when managing a patient's care plan if they are non-compliant?

   A) Enforce compliance through strict measures
   B) Understand the patient's reasons for non-compliance, involve them in their care plan, and work towards mutually agreed solutions
   C) Ignore the non-compliance and continue with the care plan as usual
   D) Restrict the patient's care options until they comply

84   How should a CNA approach a patient who is reluctant to engage in physical therapy?

   A) Insist on participation in therapy to ensure the patient follows the plan
   B) Discuss the benefits of physical therapy, address any concerns, and encourage participation while offering support
   C) Avoid physical therapy to prevent discomfort and conflict
   D) Modify the therapy plan without consulting the patient or healthcare team

85   What is the best way to communicate with a patient who has difficulty hearing?

   A) Speak loudly and use exaggerated gestures to communicate
   B) Use clear, simple language, and consider using written notes or visual aids if needed
   C) Assume the patient cannot hear and avoid engaging in conversation
   D) Provide information only to the patient's family members

86   How should a CNA handle a situation where a patient is experiencing pain after a procedure?

A) Continue with other care tasks and advise the patient to manage the pain on their own

B) Assess the patient's pain level, offer comfort measures, and report to the nurse for further instructions

C) Provide pain relief medication without authorization

D) Ignore the pain if it seems manageable and focus on other aspects of care

87 **What is the best approach to take when dealing with a patient who has specific cultural or religious needs?**

A) Ignore cultural or religious needs to focus on medical care

B) Respect and accommodate the patient's cultural or religious needs, and collaborate with the healthcare team to provide appropriate care

C) Limit care based on general practices without considering individual needs

D) Provide care as usual and avoid addressing cultural or religious concerns

88 **How should a CNA respond if a patient is exhibiting signs of a medical emergency?**

A) Document the signs and wait for scheduled medical assessments

B) Seek immediate medical assistance, provide first aid if trained, and report the situation to the healthcare team

C) Ignore the signs and continue with other care tasks

D) Provide comfort measures and wait for the healthcare team to address the emergency

89 **What is the best way to support a patient who is experiencing a change in their mental status?**

A) Avoid discussing the change to prevent distress

B) Provide reassurance, monitor the patient's mental status, and report any significant changes to the healthcare team

C) Assume the change is temporary and ignore it

D) Provide mental health resources without involving the healthcare team

90 **How should a CNA handle a situation where a patient's family member is being disruptive?**

A) Confront the family member aggressively about their behavior

B) Remain calm, address the family member's concerns respectfully, and involve the healthcare team if needed

C) Ignore the disruption and continue with care tasks

D) Ask the family member to leave the facility if their behavior continues

91 **What is the best way to manage a patient's fluid intake and output?**

A) Monitor and document fluid intake and output accurately, and report any significant changes to the healthcare team

B) Ignore fluid intake and output unless the patient complains of discomfort

C) Provide fluids without monitoring the patient's output

D) Document fluid intake and output only if the patient specifically requests

92 **How should a CNA respond if a patient expresses concerns about their discharge plan?**

A) Reassure the patient with general statements without addressing their concerns

B) Discuss the discharge plan with the patient, address their concerns, and provide information about post-discharge care

C) Avoid discussing the discharge plan to prevent further anxiety

D) Suggest the patient speak with the discharge planner for more information

93 What is the best way to provide care for a patient who is experiencing difficulty with their diet?

A) Ignore the dietary difficulties and continue with standard meal plans

B) Assess the patient's dietary needs, offer appropriate alternatives, and coordinate with the dietary department for adjustments

C) Provide standard meals without considering the patient's difficulties

D) Only address dietary needs if the patient explicitly requests changes

94 How should a CNA approach a patient who is experiencing discomfort with their environment?

A) Ignore the patient's discomfort and focus on medical care

B) Discuss the patient's concerns, make necessary adjustments to their environment, and report any issues to the appropriate personnel

C) Avoid addressing environmental concerns to prevent further discomfort

D) Suggest the patient adapt to the environment without making changes

95 What is the best way to handle a situation where a patient is experiencing difficulty with their sleep?

A) Ignore the sleep difficulties and focus on daytime care tasks

B) Assess the patient's sleep environment, offer comfort measures, and report persistent sleep issues to the healthcare team

C) Provide sleep aids without authorization

D) Advise the patient to adapt to their sleep difficulties and avoid discussing it further

96 How should a CNA respond if a patient is expressing concerns about their physical therapy progress?

A) Provide detailed explanations about their progress without involving the healthcare team

B) Discuss the patient's concerns, provide feedback on their progress, and involve the healthcare team for further evaluation if needed

C) Avoid discussing progress to prevent frustration

D) Suggest the patient focus on other aspects of their care to distract from physical therapy concerns

97 What is the best approach to take when managing a patient's care during a medical crisis?

A) Focus on immediate medical tasks and avoid communication with the patient

B) Provide essential medical care, offer reassurance, and involve the healthcare team for comprehensive management of the crisis

C) Document the crisis and wait for the healthcare team to address it

D) Provide comfort measures and wait for the patient to recover on their own

98 How should a CNA approach a patient who is feeling overwhelmed by their treatment plan?

A) Offer general reassurance and avoid discussing the treatment plan in detail

B) Provide clear, detailed information about the treatment plan, address their feelings of being overwhelmed, and offer emotional support

C) Suggest the patient focus on positive aspects to avoid feeling overwhelmed

D) Avoid discussing the treatment plan to prevent additional stress

99 What is the best way to communicate with a patient who has a speech impairment?

A) Speak loudly and use simple gestures to communicate

B) Use clear, concise language, and allow extra time for the patient to respond; consider using alternative communication methods if needed

C) Assume the patient cannot communicate and avoid engaging in conversation

D) Provide information only to the patient's family members

100 How should a CNA handle a situation where a patient is experiencing pain during a procedure?

ANSWERS

1. B)	26. B	51. B	76. B
2. B	27. B)	52. B)	77. B)
3. B	28. B	53. B	78. B
4. B	29. B	54. B	79. B)
5. B	30. B)	55. B	80. B
6. B)	31. B	56. B	81. B)
7. B	32. B	57. B	82. B
8. B	33. B)	58. B	83. B)
9. B)	34. B)	59. B	84. B)
10. B	35. B)	60. B)	85. B)
11. B	36. B	61. B	86. B)
12. B	37. B)	62. B	87. B
13. B	38. B	63. B	88. B)
14. B)	39. B	64. B)	89. B)
15. B)	40. B	65. B	90. B)
16. B	41. B	66. B)	91. B)
17. B	42. B	67. B	92. B
18. B	43. B)	68. B)	93. B
19. B)	44. B)	69. B	94. B
20. B	45. B)	70. B	95. B)
21. B	46. B	71. B)	96. B
22. B)	47. B	72. B	97. B
23. B	48. B	73. B	98. B)
24. B	49. B)	74. B	99. B
25. B)	50. B)	75. B)	

QUESTION AND ANSWERS

CHAPTHER FOUR

1 Which organization sets standards for workplace safety and health?

A) National Institutes of Health (NIH)

B) Occupational Safety and Health Administration (OSHA)

C) Centers for Disease Control and Prevention (CDC)

D) American Red Cross

2 What is the primary purpose of OSHA regulations?

A) To provide healthcare benefits

B) To ensure safe working conditions

C) To regulate medical treatments

D) To monitor patient satisfaction

3 Which of the following is a required component of a workplace safety program?

A) Patient confidentiality agreements

B) Regular safety training and drills

C) Employee performance evaluations

D) Marketing strategies

4 What should a CNA do if they encounter a hazardous spill in a patient's room?

A) Ignore it and continue working

B) Notify the housekeeping department and use proper spill containment procedures

C) Clean it up without protective equipment

D) Ask a co-worker to handle it

5 Which type of personal protective equipment (PPE) is essential when handling blood or bodily fluids?

A) Surgical mask

B) Gloves

C) Apron

D) Safety goggles

6 What does the term "universal precautions" refer to in healthcare settings?

A) Using precautions only with patients who have known infections

B) Treating all blood and body fluids as if they are infectious

C) Using precautions only during surgery

D) Isolating patients with contagious diseases

7 What is the primary focus of infection control practices?

A) To reduce patient wait times

B) To prevent the spread of infections

C) To enhance patient comfort

D) To increase healthcare worker productivity

8 **Which of the following actions should be taken to prevent the spread of infection?**

A) Frequent hand washing

B) Avoiding the use of hand sanitizer

C) Wearing the same gloves for multiple patients

D) Sharing personal protective equipment

9 **What is the purpose of a fire drill in a healthcare facility?**

A) To practice patient care techniques

B) To ensure compliance with fire safety regulations

C) To test new medical equipment

D) To assess staff productivity

10 **What should a CNA do if they discover a fire in a patient's room?**

A) Attempt to extinguish the fire alone

B) Immediately alert the fire department and follow the facility's fire evacuation plan

C) Continue providing patient care and wait for further instructions

D) Close the door and continue working

11 **What is the correct procedure for disposing of sharps?**

A) Place them in a regular trash can

B) Place them in a designated sharps container

C) Dispose of them in the biohazard waste bin

D) Flush them down the toilet

12 **What does the term "biohazard" refer to?**

A) Any item that poses a risk of infection

B) Any physical injury

C) Any hazardous chemical

D) Any medical equipment

13 **Which of the following is a key component of a safe patient handling program?**

A) Manual lifting techniques

B) Using assistive devices and proper body mechanics

C) Lifting patients without assistance

D) Avoiding the use of lifting aids

14 **What is the primary purpose of an infection control policy?**

A) To enhance patient comfort

B) To prevent the spread of infections and diseases

C) To increase staff efficiency

D) To reduce medical errors

15 **What should a CNA do if they notice a defective piece of equipment?**

A) Continue using it until it is repaired

B) Report the defect to the appropriate personnel and remove the equipment from use

C) Attempt to repair it themselves

D) Ignore the defect and use it as usual

16 What is the purpose of wearing a mask in a healthcare setting?

A) To prevent contamination from coughing or sneezing

B) To enhance patient interaction

C) To protect against physical injury

D) To improve communication with patients

17 Which of the following is a common cause of workplace injuries in healthcare settings?

A) Poor communication

B) Slip, trip, and fall accidents

C) Excessive paperwork

D) Inadequate patient records

18 What does the term "ergonomics" refer to in healthcare?

A) The study of medical equipment

B) The practice of designing work environments to fit the physical needs of workers

C) The management of patient records

D) The use of advanced medical treatments

19 What is the correct procedure for hand hygiene in a healthcare setting?

A) Wash hands for at least 20 seconds with soap and water or use an alcohol-based hand sanitizer

B) Wash hands for 10 seconds and dry with a paper towel

C) Use hand sanitizer without washing hands

D) Wash hands only when visibly soiled

20 What should be done if a CNA is exposed to a needle stick injury?

A) Ignore the injury and continue working

B) Report the incident immediately, clean the wound, and seek medical evaluation

C) Cover the injury with a bandage and continue working

D) Wait until the end of the shift to address the injury

21 What is the main goal of workplace safety regulations?

A) To ensure a pleasant work environment

B) To protect employees from injuries and illnesses

C) To increase administrative tasks

D) To monitor employee productivity

22 Which type of fire extinguisher is used for electrical fires?

A) Water extinguisher

B) Foam extinguisher

C) Carbon dioxide (CO2) extinguisher

D) Dry chemical extinguisher

23 What does the acronym "MSDS" stand for in relation to hazardous materials?

A) Material Safety Data Sheet

B) Medical Safety Documentation Sheet

C) Managed Safety Data System

D) Material Safety Delivery Sheet

24 What should be included in a facility's emergency preparedness plan?

A) Protocols for managing patient care during emergencies

B) Guidelines for employee uniforms

C) Strategies for marketing the facility

D) Plans for staff performance evaluations

25 **What is the purpose of the "R.A.C.E." acronym in fire safety?**

A) Rescue, Alarm, Contain, Evacuate

B) Rescue, Alert, Control, Extinguish

C) Rescue, Assess, Contain, Evacuate

D) React, Assess, Contain, Evacuate

26 **Which of the following is an example of a "physical hazard" in a healthcare setting?**

A) Blood borne pathogens

B) Unsafe working conditions such as wet floors

C) Stress

D) Inadequate staffing

27 **What is the purpose of using gloves in patient care?**

A) To keep hands warm

B) To prevent contamination and protect against infections

C) To enhance dexterity

D) To make tasks easier

28 **What does the term "hazardous material" include?**

A) All cleaning supplies

B) Substances that are flammable, toxic, or corrosive

C) Standard medical equipment

D) Common office supplies

29 **What should a CNA do if they experience symptoms of a work-related injury or illness?**

A) Continue working and ignore the symptoms

B) Report the symptoms to their supervisor and seek medical attention if necessary

C) Wait until the end of the shift to address the symptoms

D) Self-diagnose and treat the symptoms at home

30 **Which of the following is a key element of proper lifting techniques?**

A) Using only your back muscles to lift

B) Keeping your back straight and lifting with your legs

C) Twisting your body while lifting

D) Lifting heavy objects alone without assistance

31 **What does the "PPE" acronym stand for in healthcare?**

A) Personal Protective Equipment

B) Patient Protective Environment

C) Public Protection Equipment

D) Professional Practice Environment

32 **What is the purpose of a safety data sheet (SDS)?**

A) To provide information on how to safely handle and dispose of hazardous materials

B) To outline employee performance expectations

C) To detail patient care procedures

D) To list emergency contact numbers

33 Which of the following actions is required when handling chemical spills?

A) Ignore the spill if it is minor

B) Use appropriate personal protective equipment and follow the facility's spill response procedures

C) Clean the spill with water and continue working

D) Wait for maintenance to handle it

34 What does the acronym "BLS" stand for in emergency care?

A) Basic Life Support

B) Basic Labor Support

C) blood borne Life Safety

D) Basic Lifestyle Support

35 What is the recommended method for cleaning surfaces contaminated with bodily fluids?

A) Wipe with a dry cloth

B) Use a disinfectant that is effective against pathogens and follow proper cleaning procedures

C) Rinse with water

D) Leave the area for later cleaning

36 Which of the following is a key component of a safe patient transfer?

A) Using proper body mechanics and assistive devices

B) Lifting patients quickly to minimize discomfort

C) Transferring patients without assistance

D) Using only verbal instructions without physical support

37 What should be done if a CNA suspects a patient has a pressure ulcer?

A) Ignore it and continue with other tasks

B) Report the finding to the nurse for further assessment and documentation

C) Attempt to treat it independently

D) Document the ulcer in the CNA's personal notes

38 What is the primary purpose of an incident report?

A) To document patient care procedures

B) To record details of accidents or incidents for review and improvement

C) To track employee attendance

D) To report patient satisfaction

39 Which of the following practices helps prevent the spread of infections in a healthcare setting?

A) Using the same gloves for multiple patients

B) Following proper hand hygiene and using personal protective equipment

C) Avoiding the use of hand sanitizers

D) Sharing personal protective equipment

40 What is the primary focus of a patient safety program?

A) To enhance patient comfort

B) To prevent and minimize harm to patients during care

C) To increase staff efficiency

D) To improve facility aesthetics

41 What should a CNA do if they encounter a broken piece of equipment?

A) Continue using the equipment until it is repaired

B) Report the malfunction and remove the equipment from use immediately

C) Attempt to fix it themselves

D) Ignore the issue and use it as usual

42 Which of the following actions is appropriate for reducing the risk of falls in a healthcare facility?

A) Keeping floors clutter-free and using non-slip mats

B) Ignoring wet floors

C) Allowing patients to walk unassisted at all times

D) Using slippery rugs

43 What is the primary purpose of using isolation precautions?

A) To protect healthcare workers from injuries

B) To prevent the spread of infections from patients with contagious diseases

C) To enhance patient comfort

D) To manage patient records

44 Which of the following is a critical element of emergency response planning?

A) Knowing the location of emergency exits and equipment

B) Ignoring emergency drills

C) Focusing only on patient care

D) Avoiding the use of emergency equipment

45 What is the recommended action if a CNA notices that an emergency exit is blocked?

A) Leave it blocked until maintenance arrives

B) Report the issue immediately and ensure the exit is cleared

C) Ignore the blockage and use another exit

D) Attempt to clear the blockage themselves without reporting it

46 What is the role of a CNA in managing a patient's dietary needs?

A) Preparing and serving meals according to dietary restrictions and preferences

B) Ignoring dietary restrictions

C) Preparing meals without regard to dietary needs

D) Providing general snacks without consideration for dietary restrictions

47 Which of the following practices is essential for maintaining a safe environment for patients?

A) Regularly inspecting and maintaining equipment and facilities

B) Avoiding regular maintenance checks

C) Using outdated equipment

D) Ignoring safety protocols

48 What should a CNA do if they witness a co-worker not following safety protocols?

A) Ignore the behavior and continue working

B) Report the behavior to a supervisor or safety officer

C) Confront the co-worker in front of patients

D) Discuss the issue informally with the co-worker

49 **What is the purpose of routine safety inspections in a healthcare facility?**

A) To ensure compliance with safety regulations and identify potential hazards

B) To monitor patient satisfaction

C) To assess employee performance

D) To evaluate patient care quality

50 **Which of the following is a primary component of a safe working environment?**

A) Proper training and adherence to safety protocols

B) Minimal use of personal protective equipment

C) Ignoring safety regulations

D) Avoiding safety drills

51 **What should be done if a CNA identifies a potential safety hazard in a patient's room?**

A) Leave it as is and inform the next shift

B) Address the hazard immediately and report it to the appropriate personnel

C) Ignore it if it seems minor

D) Attempt to fix the hazard without reporting it

52 **Which of the following is a key consideration when handling patients with mobility issues?**

A) Using assistive devices and proper body mechanics

B) Relying solely on verbal instructions

C) Moving patients quickly without support

D) Avoiding the use of mobility aids

53 What should be included in a CNA's training on infection control?

A) Proper hand hygiene and use of personal protective equipment

B) How to handle non-medical tasks

C) Advanced medical procedures

D) Marketing techniques for the facility

54 What does the acronym "HICPAC" stand for in relation to infection control?

A) Healthcare Infection Control Practices Advisory Committee

B) Hospital Infection Control Practices Advisory Committee

C) Health Infection Control Procedures Advisory Committee

D) Health Infection Control and Prevention Advisory Committee

55 Which type of waste should be disposed of in a biohazard bag?

A) Non-contaminated trash

B) Paper products

C) Items contaminated with blood or bodily fluids

D) Office supplies

56 What is the recommended action if a CNA experiences a needle stick injury?

A) Continue working and ignore the injury

B) Report the incident immediately, clean the wound, and seek medical evaluation

C) Cover the injury with a bandage and continue working

D) Wait until the end of the shift to address the injury

57 What is the purpose of having a written emergency plan in a healthcare facility?

A) To ensure staff know how to respond to various emergencies

B) To enhance patient comfort

C) To improve employee performance

D) To monitor patient satisfaction

58 Which of the following is a key factor in preventing workplace violence?

A) Providing staff with training on de-escalation techniques

B) Ignoring aggressive behavior

C) Avoiding communication with patients

D) Limiting staff access to security measures

59 What should be done if a CNA notices a malfunctioning fire alarm?

A) Ignore it and continue with tasks

B) Report the malfunction immediately and ensure it is repaired

C) Attempt to fix the alarm themselves

D) Wait until the end of the shift to report it

60 What is the primary goal of safety training for CNAs?

A) To ensure that CNAs are aware of and can follow safety protocols

B) To improve patient care skills

C) To enhance administrative skills

D) To focus on time management

61 **What does the term "hazard communication" refer to?**

A) The process of informing staff about the presence of hazardous materials

B) The procedure for handling non-hazardous materials

C) The method for documenting patient care

D) The process for reporting patient complaints

62 **What is the purpose of using standard precautions in healthcare?**

A) To prevent the spread of infections regardless of the patient's known status

B) To provide specialized care for known infections

C) To focus only on high-risk patients

D) To enhance patient comfort

63 **Which of the following is an example of a chemical hazard?**

A) blood borne pathogens

B) Slip, trip, and fall accidents

C) Cleaning agents and disinfectants

D) Physical injuries

64 **What is the correct procedure for handling a fire drill?**

A) Follow the facility's fire drill procedures and evacuate calmly

B) Ignore the drill and continue working

C) Report to the fire department directly

D) Attempt to put out the fire yourself

65 What is the primary purpose of using patient restraints?

A) To prevent patients from harming themselves or others

B) To control patient movement for convenience

C) To enhance patient comfort

D) To make medical procedures easier

66 What is the recommended method for disposing of expired medications?

A) Flush them down the toilet

B) Place them in a designated medication disposal container or return them to a pharmacy

C) Throw them in the regular trash

D) Keep them in the facility's medication cabinet

67 Which of the following is a common cause of workplace injuries in healthcare settings?

A) Stress

B) Slip, trip, and fall accidents

C) Excessive paperwork

D) Poor patient care

68 What is the recommended action if a CNA encounters a patient who is agitated and aggressive?

A) Avoid engaging with the patient and leave the room

B) Use de-escalation techniques and seek assistance from a supervisor if necessary

C) Ignore the behavior and continue working

D) Confront the patient aggressively

69 **Which type of fire extinguisher is used for flammable liquids?**

A) Carbon dioxide (CO2) extinguisher

B) Water extinguisher

C) Foam extinguisher

D) Dry chemical extinguisher

70 **What is the purpose of ergonomic practices in a healthcare setting?**

A) To reduce the risk of musculoskeletal injuries and enhance worker comfort

B) To increase patient wait times

C) To improve administrative tasks

D) To enhance patient treatment procedures

☐ **Which of the following actions should be taken to prevent the spread of airborne infections?**

A) Use appropriate respiratory protection and ensure proper ventilation

B) Avoid using respiratory protection

C) Work in close proximity without protective equipment

D) Use regular masks without considering the type of infection

71 **What is the primary purpose of workplace safety signage?**

A) To provide information on hazards and safety procedures

B) To enhance the facility's appearance

C) To promote staff productivity

D) To entertain patients

72 Which of the following is an essential practice for safe patient transfer?

A) Using proper body mechanics and assistive devices

B) Lifting patients quickly without assistance

C) Ignoring patient mobility issues

D) Using outdated lifting techniques

73 What should a CNA do if they experience a work-related injury?

A) Continue working and ignore the injury

B) Report the injury to a supervisor and seek medical attention if needed

C) Self-diagnose and treat the injury independently

D) Wait until the end of the shift to address the injury

74 What is the primary goal of infection control procedures?

A) To prevent and reduce the spread of infections

B) To improve patient comfort

C) To enhance staff productivity

D) To manage facility resources

75 What does the acronym "EPA" stand for in relation to disinfectants?

A) Environmental Protection Agency

B) Emergency Protection Agency

C) Environmental Prevention Agency

D) Emergency Prevention Agency

76 **Which of the following is a key component of a disaster preparedness plan?**

A) Detailed procedures for managing various types of emergencies

B) Strategies for improving patient comfort

C) Plans for enhancing staff productivity

D) Procedures for managing facility finances

77 **What is the purpose of using a sharps container?**

A) To safely dispose of needles, blades, and other sharp objects

B) To store general waste

C) To keep medical supplies organized

D) To dispose of food waste

78 **What should be done if a CNA is exposed to a potentially infectious material?**

A) Continue working and monitor for symptoms

B) Report the exposure immediately, follow facility protocols, and seek medical evaluation

C) Ignore the exposure and seek medical help only if symptoms appear

D) Document the exposure and address it later

79 **Which of the following actions is important for preventing needle-stick injuries?**

A) Disposing of needles immediately in a sharps container

B) Recapping needles after use

C) Placing needles in regular trash

D) Handling needles with bare hands

80 **What is the primary focus of safety audits in healthcare facilities?**

A) To identify and address potential safety hazards

B) To evaluate patient satisfaction

C) To monitor staff performance

D) To review patient care records

81 **Which of the following is an example of a biological hazard?**

A) Infected bodily fluids

B) Slippery floors

C) Broken equipment

D) Unsafe working conditions

82 **What should be done if a CNA encounters a chemical spill in a patient's room?**

A) Clean it up without protective equipment

B) Report the spill immediately and follow the facility's chemical spill procedures

C) Ignore the spill and wait for maintenance

D) Use a wet cloth to clean the spill

83 **What is the primary goal of workplace ergonomics?**

A) To reduce the risk of musculoskeletal injuries

B) To improve patient satisfaction

C) To increase administrative tasks

D) To enhance facility aesthetics

84 **What does the term "clean technique" refer to in infection control?**

A) Using standard procedures to minimize the risk of infection

B) Sterilizing equipment for invasive procedures

C) Using antiseptics to clean wounds

D) Disinfecting surfaces and equipment

85 **What should a CNA do if they identify a potential safety hazard in the workplace?**

A) Ignore it and continue working

B) Report the hazard to the appropriate personnel and take corrective action if possible

C) Attempt to fix it themselves without reporting

D) Wait until the end of the shift to address it

86 **What is the purpose of emergency preparedness training for CNAs?**

A) To ensure staff are equipped to respond effectively to emergencies

B) To focus solely on patient care techniques

C) To improve administrative skills

D) To monitor patient satisfaction

87 **Which of the following is a key aspect of proper infection control in patient care?**

A) Using personal protective equipment and practicing good hand hygiene

B) Ignoring standard precautions

C) Avoiding the use of antiseptics

D) Using shared personal protective equipment

88 **What is the primary function of safety drills in a healthcare facility?**

A) To prepare staff for emergency situations and ensure they can respond effectively

B) To improve patient comfort

C) To increase staff productivity

D) To assess patient satisfaction

89 **What should a CNA do if they encounter a broken safety device?**

A) Continue using it until it is repaired

B) Report the malfunction immediately and remove the device from use

C) Attempt to repair it themselves

D) Ignore the issue and use it as usual

ANSWERS

1. B)	19. B	37. B)	55. C)	73. A)
2. A	20. B)	38. B)	56. B)	74. B)
3. B	21. B	39. B)	57. A)	75. A)
4. A)	22. A	40. B)	58. A)	76. A)
5. B)	23. B)	41. B)	59. B)	77. A)
6. B	24. B	42. A)	60. A)	78. A)
7. B	25. B)	43. B)	61. A)	79. B)
8. B	26. B	44. A)	62. A)	80. A)
9. A)	27. B).	45. B)	63. C)	81. A)
10. B)	28. B)	46. A)	64. A)	82. A)
11. B)	29. A)	47. A)	65. A)	83. B)
12. B)	30. A)	48. B)	66. B).	84. A)
13. B)	31. B)	49. A)	67. B)	85. A)
14. A)	32. B)	50. A)	68. B)	86. B)
15. B)	33. A).	51. B)	69. D)	87. A)
16. B	34. B)	52. A)	70. A)	88. A)
17. A)	35. B)	53. A)	71. A)	89. A)
18. B	36. A).	54. A)	72. A)	90. B)

QUESTION AND ANSWERS

CHAPTER FIVE

1 **What is the best way to begin preparing for the CNA exam?**

A) Skim through random study materials

B) Review the exam content outline and study guide

C) Watch television for relaxation

D) Rely solely on practice exams

2 **Which of the following should be the focus of your study plan?**

A) Memorizing all textbook content

B) Understanding key concepts and procedures

C) Avoiding practice questions

D) Reading unrelated materials

3 **What type of study resource is most effective for learning hands-on skills?**

A) Textbooks

B) Video demonstrations and simulations

C) Online forums

D) Fiction books

4 **How often should you review material to retain information effectively?**

A) Once, the day before the exam

B) Regularly, with spaced repetition

C) Only when you feel like studying

D) Sporadically, without a schedule

5 **What is a good strategy for taking practice exams?**

A) Take them only once

B) Use them to identify weak areas and focus on those

C) Skip them entirely

D) Rely on them as your only study method

6 **Which of the following is a key area of focus for the CNA written exam?**

A) Understanding medical terminology

B) Cooking techniques

C) Sports history

D) Art appreciation

7 **How should you approach studying for the clinical skills portion of the CNA exam?**

A) Study clinical skills theoretically only

B) Practice skills with a partner or in a lab setting

C) Focus on multiple-choice questions only

D) Rely on online videos without hands-on practice

8 **What is important to remember when taking the CNA written exam?**

A) You can skip questions and return to them later

B) Read each question carefully and manage your time

C) Answer questions based on your first guess only

D) Focus on speed over accuracy

9 **How can you reduce test anxiety before the CNA exam?**

A) Cram the night before

B) Maintain a regular study schedule and practice relaxation techniques

C) Avoid studying completely

D) Ignore the exam format and practice randomly

10 **What should you bring with you on the day of the CNA exam?**

A) Only a pencil

B) Required identification and any materials specified by the testing center

C) A large bag of study materials

D) Snacks and drinks

11 **What is the purpose of the CNA skills test?**

A) To assess your ability to perform specific healthcare tasks

B) To evaluate your knowledge of medical history

C) To test your ability to memorize information

D) To measure your reading speed

12 **Which of the following is an example of a common clinical skill tested in the CNA exam?**

A) Administering medications

B) Taking vital signs

C) Designing care plans

D) Performing advanced surgeries

13 **What type of questions are typically found on the CNA written exam?**

A) True or false

B) Multiple choice

C) Essay

D) Fill-in-the-blank

14 **What is a good method for memorizing medical terminology?**

A) Flashcards and repetition

B) Reading only once

C) Ignoring terminology

D) Memorizing entire chapters

15 **How can you best prepare for situational judgment questions on the CNA exam?**

A) Practice scenarios and review best practices for patient care

B) Guess based on intuition

C) Ignore situational questions

D) Focus only on theoretical knowledge

16 **What is one effective way to manage time during the CNA exam?**

A) Spend equal time on each question

B) Allocate more time to questions you find difficult

C) Rush through all questions quickly

D) Skip questions and come back to them at the end

17 **How important is it to understand the CNA exam format before taking the test?**

A) It is essential for effective preparation and performance

B) It is not necessary; the content is more important

C) It only matters for the written exam

D) It is less important than studying individual topics

18 **What should you do if you encounter a question on the exam that you do not know?**

A) Leave it blank

B) Make an educated guess based on what you know

C) Spend excessive time on it

D) Skip it and do not revisit

19 **How can group study sessions be beneficial for CNA exam preparation?**

A) They allow for discussion and clarification of difficult concepts

B) They are a waste of time

C) They can lead to confusion and distractions

D) They replace individual study needs

20 **What is the best way to handle a mistake made during the CNA skills test?**

A) Panic and worry about the result

B) Stay calm, correct the mistake if possible, and continue with the test

C) Ignore it and proceed without addressing the error

D) Complain to the proctor

21 **Which study technique is often recommended for retaining detailed information?**

A) Re-reading the same material multiple times

B) Summarizing information and teaching it to others

C) Skipping difficult sections

D) Focusing only on the easiest topics

22 **What role do practice tests play in CNA exam preparation?**

A) They help gauge your knowledge and identify areas needing improvement

B) They are less important than reviewing textbooks

C) They are only useful for relaxing before the exam

D) They replace the need for any other study materials

23 **How should you prepare for questions related to patient rights and ethics?**

A) Study relevant guidelines and case scenarios

B) Skip these topics as they are not important

C) Only focus on clinical skills

D) Rely on general knowledge without specific study

24 **What is an effective strategy for answering multiple-choice questions on the CNA exam?**

A) Eliminate obviously incorrect answers and choose the best option

B) Guess randomly

C) Choose the longest answer

D) Select the first answer you see

25 How can you use study guides effectively for CNA exam preparation?

A) Follow them closely and use them to structure your study plan

B) Use them as a secondary resource only

C) Ignore them and focus on other materials

D) Read them once and forget about them

26 What is a good approach to understanding and remembering procedures?

A) Practice them repeatedly in a hands-on setting

B) Read about them once and move on

C) Memorize the steps without practicing

D) Focus only on written descriptions

27 How should you approach studying for the CNA exam if you have limited time?

A) Prioritize the most important topics and practice key skills

B) Try to cover every topic equally

C) Focus solely on practice exams

D) Skip studying and rely on test-taking skills

28 Which type of study environment is most conducive to effective learning?

A) A quiet and organized space with minimal distractions

B) A noisy and chaotic environment

C) A space with constant interruptions

D) Studying in a public place with lots of activity

29 **What is the benefit of using flashcards for studying medical terms and procedures?**

A) They help with memorization through active recall and repetition

B) They are not very useful

C) They only cover a small portion of the material

D) They are a waste of time

30 **How should you use feedback from practice exams in your study plan?**

A) Address any weaknesses and adjust your study focus accordingly

B) Ignore feedback and continue with the same study plan

C) Focus only on questions you got wrong

D) Rely on feedback for practice exams only

31 **Which resource is typically used to understand the format of the CNA skills test?**

A) The CNA test handbook or guide provided by the certification body

B) General textbooks on healthcare

C) Online forums and blogs

D) Non-medical books

32 **What is the importance of understanding patient care protocols in the CNA exam?**

A) They are crucial for providing safe and effective patient care

B) They are not relevant to the exam

C) They only matter for the clinical portion

D) They are less important than medical terminology

33 **What should you do if you encounter an unfamiliar procedure during the clinical skills test?**

A) Ask the proctor for clarification

B) Perform the procedure as best as you can based on your training

C) Skip the procedure and focus on other tasks

D) Panic and become overwhelmed

34 **How can you effectively use mnemonic devices for the CNA exam?**

A) To help remember complex information and lists

B) To replace studying entirely

C) To memorize only the easiest concepts

D) To focus on irrelevant details

35 **Which type of practice questions are most beneficial for the CNA written exam?**

A) Questions that mimic the format and difficulty of the actual exam

B) Random questions from unrelated topics

C) Questions without answers or explanations

D) Multiple-choice questions without any practice

36 **What should you do if you are unsure about an answer during the CNA written exam?**

A) Use elimination strategies to narrow down choices

B) Leave it blank and move on

C) Choose the first answer that seems right

D) Skip it without further consideration

37 **What role does regular review play in preparing for the CNA exam?**

A) It reinforces learning and helps with long-term retention

B) It is not necessary if you study once

C) It only applies to theoretical knowledge

D) It is less important than practicing skills

38 **How can you ensure you are familiar with the CNA exam's practical component?**

A) Participate in hands-on practice and simulations

B) Focus solely on theoretical study

C) Avoid practicing procedures

D) Study only written material

39 **What is the benefit of joining a study group for CNA exam preparation?**

A) It provides support, diverse perspectives, and accountability

B) It can be a distraction

C) It is not necessary for successful preparation

D) It only benefits those who are already well-prepared

40 **How important is it to review state-specific regulations and guidelines for the CNA exam?**

A) Very important, as they may be included in the exam

B) Not important at all

C) Only important for clinical skills

D) Less important than general knowledge

41 **What should you focus on when studying patient safety practices?**

A) Proper techniques for preventing accidents and ensuring patient safety

B) General safety tips unrelated to healthcare

C) Only theoretical knowledge without practical application

D) Ignoring patient safety practices

42 **How can you effectively use study guides for preparing for the CNA exam?**

A) Use them to structure your study sessions and focus on key areas

B) Only read through them without practicing

C) Ignore them and rely on other resources

D) Use them as a final review only

43 **What is a common format for questions on the CNA written exam?**

A) Multiple choice with one correct answer

B) True/false statements only

C) Essay questions

D) Fill-in-the-blank questions only

44 **How should you approach studying for both the written and clinical portions of the CNA exam?**

A) Balance your study time between theoretical knowledge and hands-on practice

B) Focus solely on one portion at a time

C) Study only for the portion you find easier

D) Ignore one portion and only study for the other

45 **What is a recommended strategy for dealing with test-taking stress?**

A) Practice relaxation techniques and maintain a positive mindset

B) Avoid preparation to reduce stress

C) Focus only on test anxiety without addressing study needs

D) Ignore stress and rely solely on test-taking skills

46 **How can you use previous exam takers' experiences to aid in your preparation?**

A) Learn from their tips and insights about the exam format and content

B) Rely solely on their experiences without studying yourself

C) Ignore their experiences and focus only on your own study methods

D) Only consider their experiences if they had high scores

47 **What should you include in your study routine to prepare effectively for the CNA exam?**

A) Regular review, practice exams, and hands-on skills practice

B) Random studying without a plan

C) Only reading textbook chapters

D) Relying solely on last-minute cramming

48 **How can you ensure that you are up-to-date with the latest CNA exam requirements?**

A) Review the latest guidelines and requirements from the certifying body

B) Rely on outdated information

C) Focus only on historical exam formats

D) Ignore updates and rely on previous knowledge

49 What should you do if you have difficulty understanding a specific topic?

A) Seek additional resources or ask for help from instructors or peers

B) Skip the topic and focus on easier material

C) Avoid studying the difficult topic

D) Guess on exam questions related to the topic

50 How can you effectively utilize online resources for CNA exam preparation?

A) Use reputable sources and practice questions relevant to the exam

B) Rely solely on online forums without verifying accuracy

C) Use random online materials without checking credibility

D) Focus only on non-interactive resources

51 What is a good method for reviewing clinical skills before the CNA exam?

A) Practice with a partner or in a clinical skills lab

B) Read descriptions of skills without practicing

C) Watch videos without hands-on practice

D) Ignore clinical skills review

52 How should you prepare for questions on patient care and communication?

A) Study scenarios and best practices for effective communication and patient care

B) Focus only on technical skills

C) Ignore patient care aspects

D) Rely solely on textbook definitions

53 What role does understanding patient privacy and confidentiality play in the CNA exam?

A) It is crucial for both the written and clinical portions of the exam

B) It is not relevant to the exam

C) It only matters for the clinical portion

D) It is less important than other topics

54 How can you improve your test-taking skills for the CNA exam?

A) Practice with timed exams and review test-taking strategies

B) Rely solely on your current skills without practice

C) Avoid practicing under exam conditions

D) Focus only on memorization

55 What is a helpful approach to studying patient care procedures?

A) Break procedures down into steps and practice each step

B) Memorize procedures without understanding

C) Focus only on theoretical aspects

D) Ignore procedural practice

56 How can you use study schedules to enhance your preparation for the CNA exam?

A) Create a detailed plan and allocate time for each topic and practice

B) Study randomly without a schedule

C) Focus only on last-minute reviews

D) Avoid planning and study as you go

57 What is an effective way to address knowledge gaps discovered during practice exams?

A) Focus additional study time on the areas where you are weak

B) Ignore the gaps and focus on stronger areas

C) Only practice with new questions

D) Rely solely on practice exams without additional study

58 How should you approach the review of patient rights and ethics for the CNA exam?

A) Study relevant guidelines and ethical considerations in patient care

B) Focus only on technical skills

C) Skip this topic as it is less important

D) Rely solely on intuition

59 What is a good practice for using practice questions effectively?

A) Review both correct and incorrect answers to understand reasoning

B) Only focus on questions you answered incorrectly

C) Skip reviewing answers and focus on taking more questions

D) Use practice questions as a sole study method

60 How can you make the most out of CNA exam review sessions?

A) Actively engage in review, discuss with peers, and clarify doubts

B) Passively listen without interaction

C) Avoid participating and focus on individual study

D) Only review what you already know

61 **What should be your focus when preparing for the clinical skills portion of the CNA exam?**

A) Mastering hands-on skills and demonstrating them correctly

B) Memorizing written descriptions of skills

C) Focusing only on theoretical knowledge

D) Avoiding practice and relying on test-taking strategies

62 **How important is it to understand the different types of CNA exam questions?**

A) Very important for effectively answering and managing time during the exam

B) Not important; focus only on content

C) Only important for the clinical portion

D) Less important than practicing skills

63 **What should you do if you feel overwhelmed during your exam preparation?**

A) Take breaks, seek support, and adjust your study plan

B) Continue studying without breaks

C) Ignore the feeling and push through

D) Avoid studying until you feel better

64 **What is a common pitfall to avoid when preparing for the CNA exam?**

A) Over-reliance on one study method or resource

B) Using diverse study materials and methods

C) Practicing regularly and reviewing frequently

D) Taking practice exams to assess progress

65   How can you ensure you are well-prepared for the patient care scenarios in the CNA exam?

A) Study common scenarios and review best practices for patient interactions

B) Focus only on clinical skills

C) Ignore patient care scenarios

D) Memorize patient care protocols without understanding

66   What is the best way to approach studying for a comprehensive exam like the CNA exam?

A) Break down the material into manageable sections and review regularly

B) Cram all material in one session

C) Focus on one topic at a time without review

D) Skip difficult sections

67   How can using flashcards assist in preparing for the CNA exam?

A) They help with memorization of key terms and concepts through active recall

B) They are not useful for CNA exam preparation

C) They should be used only for last-minute review

D) They are only helpful for memorizing definitions

68   What is a good practice for maintaining focus during study sessions?

A) Set specific goals and take regular breaks to stay engaged

B) Study for long hours without breaks

C) Study in a distracting environment

D) Focus only on one topic at a time

69 **How should you use feedback from instructors or peers to enhance your exam preparation?**

A) Incorporate feedback into your study plan and address areas for improvement

B) Ignore feedback and continue with your existing plan

C) Focus only on feedback about strengths

D) Use feedback as a secondary resource

70 **What is a key factor in effectively preparing for the CNA clinical skills test?**

A) Practicing skills in a realistic setting and receiving feedback

B) Reading about skills without practice

C) Focusing only on the written exam

D) Memorizing steps without understanding

71 **What should you do if you are unsure how to perform a specific skill on the clinical test?**

A) Perform the skill to the best of your ability based on training

B) Skip the skill and move on

C) Ask the proctor for help

D) Panic and become overwhelmed

72 **What role do study aids such as diagrams and charts play in preparing for the CNA exam?**

A) They provide visual aids that help in understanding and memorizing concepts

B) They are less important than text-based resources

C) They should be avoided in favor of written materials

D) They are only useful for visual learners

73 **How can practicing with a study partner benefit your exam preparation?**

A) It allows for discussion, clarification of concepts, and mutual support

B) It can lead to distractions and less focus

C) It is only beneficial if your partner is an expert

D) It should be avoided to focus on solo study

74 **What is a common strategy for managing time during the CNA written exam?**

A) Allocate time based on the difficulty of each question and review if time permits

B) Spend equal time on each question regardless of difficulty

C) Rush through questions to finish quickly

D) Skip questions you find difficult

75 **How should you use a CNA exam study guide effectively?**

A) Follow it systematically to cover all relevant topics and practice areas

B) Use it as a secondary resource

C) Only refer to it once before the exam

D) Skip it in favor of other materials

76 What should you do if you encounter difficulty with patient care techniques?

A) Seek additional resources or assistance and practice regularly

B) Avoid practicing these techniques

C) Rely solely on theoretical knowledge

D) Ignore the difficulty and move on

77 How can you best utilize your study time in the weeks leading up to the CNA exam?

A) Create a structured schedule and review all key areas consistently

B) Study sporadically without a plan

C) Focus only on new material

D) Rely on last-minute cramming

78 What is a useful way to review patient care and safety procedures?

A) Practice procedures and review best practices regularly

B) Memorize procedures without understanding their application

C) Focus solely on theoretical knowledge

D) Avoid reviewing procedures

79 How can reviewing past practice test results help in your exam preparation?

A) It helps identify strengths and weaknesses to focus study efforts

B) It is not useful if you have already reviewed the material

C) It only helps if you scored high on practice tests

D) It should be done only once

80 What is the best approach to understanding and retaining complex information for the CNA exam?

A) Break down information into smaller parts and use active learning techniques

B) Read through material passively

C) Memorize without understanding

D) Focus only on easier topics

81 How should you prepare for questions on infection control procedures?

A) Study standard protocols and best practices for infection prevention

B) Focus only on general health topics

C) Ignore infection control procedures

D) Rely on theoretical knowledge only

82 What is the importance of practicing with simulation tests for the CNA exam?

A) It helps familiarize you with the exam format and question types

B) It is less important than reading textbooks

C) It should be used only as a secondary resource

D) It is not necessary if you study other materials

83 What is a good strategy for answering multiple-choice questions on the CNA exam?

A) Eliminate incorrect options and choose the best answer

B) Choose answers based on intuition only

C) Select the first option you see

D) Skip questions you are unsure about

84 **How can you ensure you are prepared for the clinical skills portion of the CNA exam?**

A) Practice skills frequently and review procedures in detail

B) Focus only on the written exam

C) Memorize steps without practicing

D) Ignore practical skills review

85 **What is a recommended study habit for retaining information effectively?**

A) Regular review and active engagement with the material

B) Cramming the night before

C) Focusing on only one topic at a time

D) Relying on passive reading

86 **How should you manage your study time when preparing for the CNA exam?**

A) Create a balanced study schedule that covers all topics

B) Study only when you feel like it

C) Focus on one topic intensively at the expense of others

D) Study in short, irregular sessions

87 **What is the benefit of discussing exam content with peers or instructors?**

A) It provides clarity, diverse perspectives, and reinforces understanding

B) It can lead to confusion and misinformation

C) It is less beneficial than studying alone

D) It should be avoided to focus on individual study

88 What should you do if you feel unprepared as the exam date approaches?

A) Adjust your study plan, seek additional resources, and review key areas

B) Panic and avoid studying further

C) Skip reviewing difficult topics

D) Rely solely on last-minute cramming

89 What is a useful technique for memorizing key procedures and protocols?

A) Practice regularly and use mnemonic devices

B) Read through material once and forget it

C) Focus only on theoretical descriptions

D) Avoid memorization

90 How can you improve your understanding of complex topics in the CNA exam?

A) Break them down into simpler parts and use various study resources

B) Memorize complex topics without understanding

C) Skip difficult topics

D) Focus only on easier material

91 What should be your focus when studying patient care techniques?

A) Mastering the application and understanding best practices

B) Memorizing descriptions without practice

C) Ignoring patient care techniques

D) Focusing only on theoretical aspects

92 **What is a good approach for dealing with difficult questions during the CNA exam?**

A) Use logical reasoning and elimination strategies

B) Skip them without attempting

C) Guess randomly

D) Focus on them exclusively

93 **How can you use mock exams to prepare for the CNA exam effectively?**

A) To simulate the exam environment and assess your readiness

B) To only review incorrect answers

C) To focus solely on multiple-choice questions

D) To replace all other forms of study

94 **What is important to remember when reviewing patient care documentation?**

A) Understand the importance of accurate and clear documentation

B) Focus only on how to fill out forms

C) Ignore documentation practices

D) Rely solely on theoretical knowledge

95 **How can you prepare for questions on ethical dilemmas in patient care?**

A) Study ethical guidelines and review case studies

B) Ignore ethics and focus on clinical skills

C) Rely only on personal opinions

D) Memorize ethical terms without understanding

ANSWERS

1. A)	**25. A)**	49. A)	73. A)
2. A)	26. A)	50. A)	74. A)
3. A)	27. A)	51. A)	75. A)
4. A)	28. A)	52. A)	76. A)
5. A)	29. A)	53. A)	77. A)
6. A)	30. A)	54. A)	78. A)
7. A)	31. A)	55. A)	79. A)
8. A)	32. A)	56. A)	80. A)
9. A)	33. A)	57. A)	81. A)
10. A)	34. A)	58. A)	82. A)
11. A)	35. A)	59. A)	83. A)
12. A)	36. A)	60. A)	84. A)
13. A)	37. A)	61. A)	85. A)
14. A)	38. A)	62. A)	86. A)
15. A)	39. A)	**63. A)**	87. A)
16. A)	40. A)	64. A)	88. A)
17. A)	41. A)	65. A)	**89. A)**
18. A)	42. A)	66. A)	90. A)
19. A)	43. A)	67. A)	91. A)
20. A)	44. A)	68. A)	92. A)
21. A)	45. A)	69. A)	93. A)
22. A)	46. A)	70. A)	94. A)
23. A)	**47. A)**	71. A)	95. A)
24. A)	48. A)	72. A)	96. A)